LaUSen

Michael van Straten

super

radiance

detox

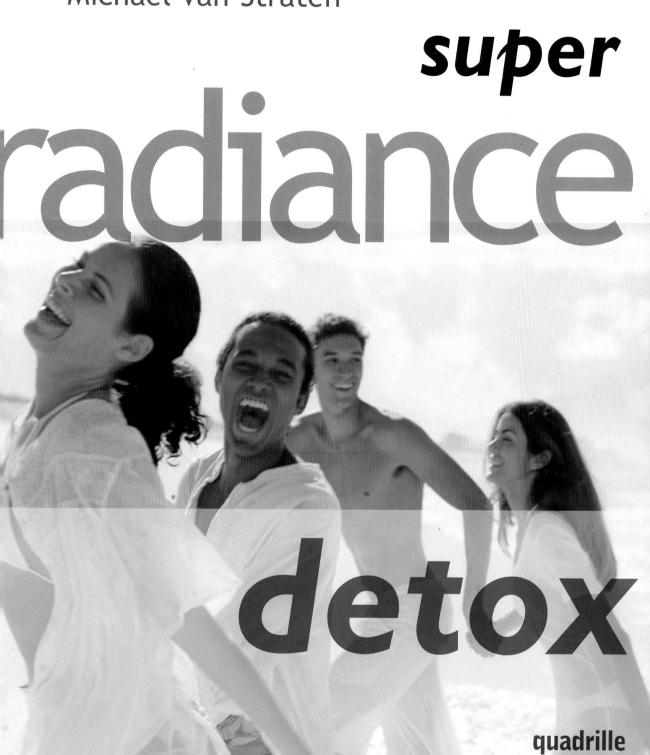

quadrille

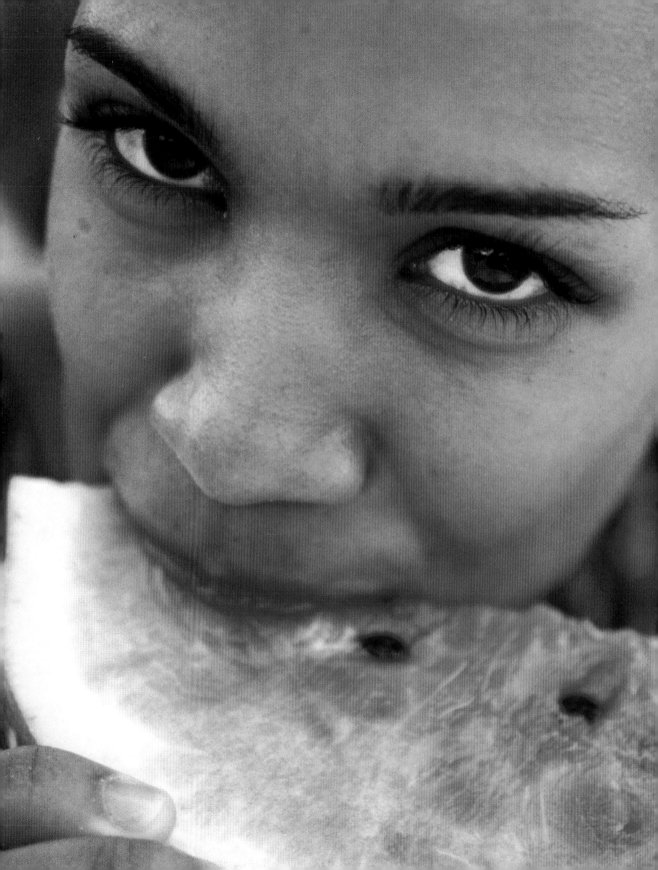

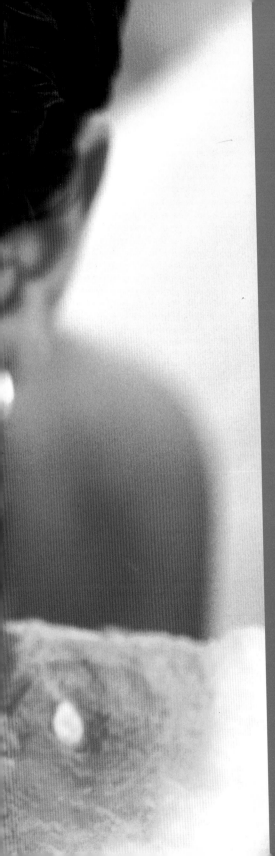

contents

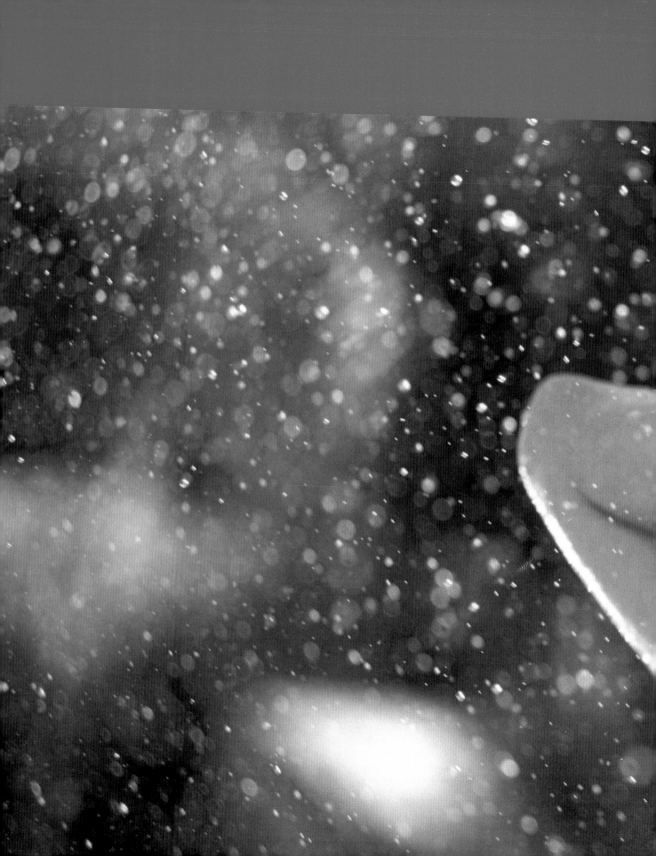

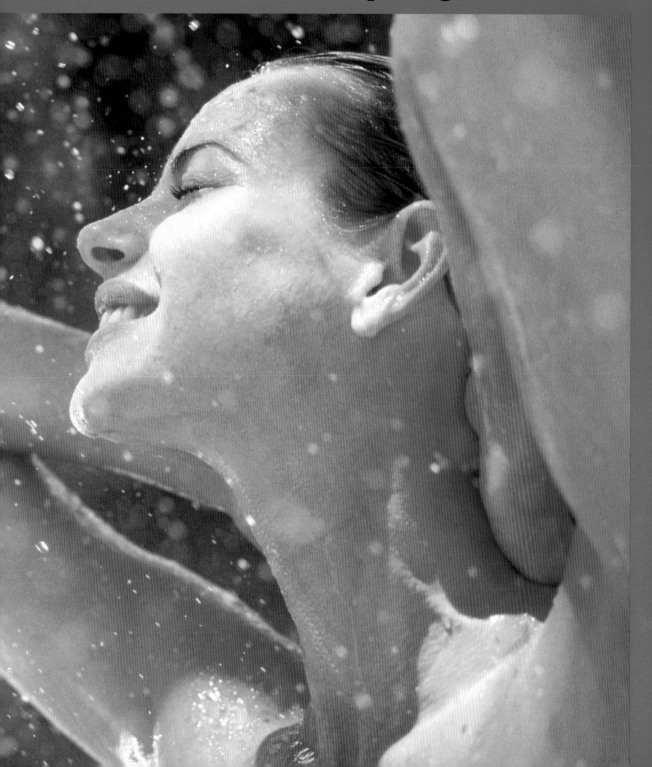

part 1 the detox programmes

the search for super radiance

'It looks good, tastes good and by golly it does you good' may be one of the great advertising slogans of all time, but there's a lot of truth in it, just as there is in the saying 'You are what you eat'. This is especially the case when it comes to radiance.

People imagine that to be radiant, you have to be young and beautiful, but this is far from the truth. Radiance has nothing to do with the conventional perception of 'beauty'. No-one could describe Mrs Ghandi, the late prime minister of India, as a beauty, but I sat next to her once at a small private dinner and she positively oozed radiance.

The truth is that to look radiant on the outside you have to be radiant on the inside. It's the combination of both that results in super radiance. It shows in healthy skin, hair and nails, but it comes from general good health, good bowel function, strong bones and pain-free joints and you can achieve all these by eating the right things and clearing all the rubbish out of your system.

So if you've looked in the mirror and think you're sliding down the radiance scale, now's the time to take control, start your detox for radiance plan and change your eating habits for good. Simple changes can not only stop the clock, but can even turn it back.

If your idea of cooking is ready meals from the freezer to the microwave, instant soups, pot noodles and take-away kebabs, then you shouldn't be surprised if your skin looks less than radiant. People forget that skin is one of the body's major organs of elimination and many of the waste products and irritant materials that result from the chemical factory that makes up your daily metabolism, find their way to the outside world through this delicate membrane. Efficient elimination of bodily waste will also be hampered by constipation, which is a frequent cause of dull and lifeless skin. It's also uncomfortable and can produce painful wind and unsightly bloating, which in turn makes it difficult to wear any clothes that fit snugly round the waist. Proper detoxing and long-term changes to your eating patterns can solve even a lifetime of constipation and will enable you to live without the bowel-irritating effects of laxatives.

Excessive amounts of alcohol and caffeine may also be implicated as the cause of some skin problems. These are both vasoconstrictors – they narrow the tiny blood capillaries at the end of the circulatory system – and can restrict the flow of vital nutrients to the skin

In addition, protecting your joints, ligaments and muscles is a must as there is nothing as certain as pain to dull your natural radiance. Similarly, you need protection from degenerative diseases like arthritis and osteoporosis, and to ward off heart disease, strokes and cancer. Again, what you eat has a bearing on all of this, and once you have got into the regular habit of detoxing to keep the chemical load to a minimum, you must restructure your everyday eating to include all of the most essential foods.

And finally, don't forget that environmental pollution, pregnancy, stress, anxiety, depression, menstruation, thyroid problems, the menopause and, of course, smoking, can all play their part in denying you the radiance you deserve.

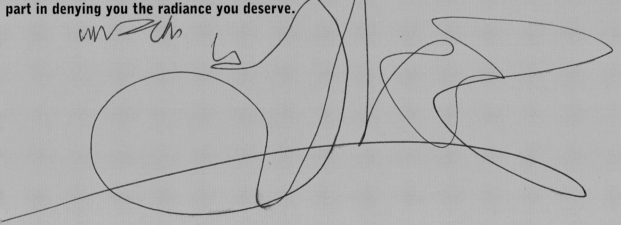

getting your radiance back on track

So what do you need to eat to get your radiance back on track? First of all, being seriously ill does nothing for your radiance so you should eat foods that protect from illness and disease. Believe it or not, prunes are top of the list, with the highest protective content of any food, so you should eat three every day. Cabbages, blueberries, Brazil nuts, shellfish and pumpkin seeds are rich sources of selenium and zinc and of cancer-protective plant chemicals, while wholegrain cereals are your best protection against bowel cancer, watercress protects the lungs, and tomatoes are rich in lycopene, which helps prevent hormone-linked cancers.

Stave off arthritis by eating oily fish three times a week and drink at least a quarter of a litre of soya milk, or eat a portion of tofu or soya beans each day, as these contain plant hormones that counteract the problems of the menopause and protect against osteoporosis.

Other essential foods – full of vitamins and skin-protective enzymes – are tropical fruits like pineapple, mango, kiwi, papaya and passion fruit, and don't forget spinach, kale and pak choi, for their antioxidants and carotenoids – also good for eyesight. There's nothing worse for crow's feet than straining to read! And while we're talking fruit and vegetables, eat lots of cherries and strawberries for their vitamin C and the essential bioflavonoids that protect the tiniest blood vessels and prevent unsightly thread veins.

And last but not least, get your oats every day from porridge or muesli. Oats are a great de-stressing food and less stress means fewer wrinkles. They also contain silicon – important for the collagen that fills out the shape of your face.

Then there are three nutrients that are absolutely vital for healthy skin. Any deficiencies of these will quickly be reflected in your appearance.

vitamin A

This is necessary for the building of new skin tissue and to heal skin damage. Fortunately, your body is clever enough to manufacture vitamin A from betacarotene, so make sure you eat an average portion from this list every single day – liver (not if you're pregnant), carrots, spinach, broccoli, sweet potatoes, cantaloupe melon, nectarines and dried apricots. You may be surprised to know that a vegetarian curry of yams, carrots, sweet potatoes, peas, sweetcorn, broccoli and spinach, will give you just about twice as much vitamin A as you need for one day.

vitamin E

The super-radiance nutrient that's so important for the health of the skin and as a protective antioxidant. Get your daily requirements by eating avocados, asparagus, extra-virgin olive oil, cod-liver oil, wheatgerm oil, sunflower seeds and almonds. In fact, the avocado is nature's gift to the skin because as well as containing vitamin E, it is an excellent source of B vitamins, a good source of iron and phosphorous, the second highest fruit source of pantothenic acid, which is essential for healthy skin and nails and is rich in the protein glutathione – a powerful antioxidant that protects your skin from ageing. But it is its monounsaturated fat content which is of particular importance, as it plays a major role in helping your body to get rid of cholesterol.

zinc

Make sure that your complement of zinc is up to the mark too by adding red meat, shellfish, sardines, poultry, kidney beans and pumpkin seeds to your shopping list. By the way, zinc is also vital for the manufacture of sperm. The richest source of all is the oyster – Casanova was reputed to eat seventy a day!

deal with those skin problems

A diet that consists mostly of processed, packaged and convenience foods is more likely to cause skin problems than one that is largely made up of fresh foods. Convenience foods are not only deficient in the essential nutrients, but are also likely to contain large amounts of sugar, salt, saturated fats and potentially allergenic substances in the form of colourings, preservatives and flavourings. For example, foods or drinks containing the yellow colouring tartrazine, E102, may aggravate eczema or cause urticaria and the emulsifiers and stabilizers, E430 and E431, are another eczema irritant. In the same way, the benzoate preservatives, E218 and E219, and the fungicide, hexamine, E239, can all cause skin irritation.

But while eczema may be triggered by an allergic reaction to some additives, other foods may be suspect as well, so you need to choose your skin-nutrient-rich foods with care. Many eczema sufferers may react badly to dairy products, shellfish, nuts or seeds, all of which are common allergens in sensitive individuals. And citrus fruits and very hot and spicy dishes – some spices like chillies have irritant properties – are also often triggers for eczema. So it's only common sense to make sure that you take account of any of your own personal allergic reactions before making major changes to your eating habits.

And finally, as many teenagers know to their cost, burgers, chips and chocolate will make their acne worse than ever. Most dermatologists do not believe this to be true, but a diet rich in fats and sugars increases the elimination of fatty acids through the skin. These then attract dirt and bacteria which become locked inside the sebaceous glands where they multiply and cause the unsightly and painful zits of acne.

deal with those hair problems

Many factors can affect the health of your crowning glory, but most of them can be improved by paying more careful attention to what you eat. Most important for radiant hair are fruit, vegetables and salads, all of which give you beta-carotene and vitamin C; wholemeal bread, brown rice and oats for vitamin B; oily fish for Omega-3 fatty acids and vitamin D; shellfish and pumpkin seeds for zinc; liver, dates, dried apricots, raisins and prunes for iron; low-fat dairy products for calcium; brazil nuts for selenium; olive oil and safflower oil for polyunsaturates; avocados, sunflower-seed oil, natural, unsalted peanut butter for vitamin E, and eggs for cysteine and methionine.

All women lose some hair as they get older, and after the menopause it tends to become finer and thinner. Women also frequently suffer hair loss two or three months after childbirth, but it soon regrows. For both men and women, anaemia can trigger hair loss, though this is more common in women, especially those who suffer from heavy periods. If you're anaemic, more iron-rich foods will help.

deal with those nail problems

Contrary to popular belief, nails aren't made of calcium but of a horny material called keratin, and they grow from the root end at a speed of roughly 1mm a week. To encourage strong nails and healthy growth, you need complex B vitamins, zinc plus pantothenic acid – remember, there's a rich supply of pantothenic acid in avocados – together, of course, with a generally sensible and healthy diet.

Most people think that white spots on the nails are a sign of calcium deficiency, but in fact they're nearly always caused by a lack of zinc – eat a handful of pumpkin seeds every day for a supply of this essential mineral. Shellfish are another enormously rich source of zinc, and best of all are oysters, as long as you're not allergic to them. But if you love them, it's a good excuse to indulge your passion.

One of the traditional foods for healthy nails is gelatin, which you can now get as a special nail-formula capsule. And last but not least, eat garlic. This amazing little bulb has powerful anti-fungal properties – perfect for those unsightly fungal nail infections.

time to detox?

Dull blotchy skin, lifeless hair, breaking fingernails, early wrinkles, cellulite and a total absence of radiance can be the result of poor nutrition, external toxic damage from too much sun, smoking and environmental pollution, or an internal accumulation of waste products. Your radiance can also be affected by too much booze. This is not only damaging on its own, but also interferes with your body's ability to absorb nutrients. Any chronic digestive disease can also do this and thyroid problems, long-term illness, pain and the side effects of medication can all be equally damaging. Answer the Super Radiance quiz now to learn just how much you need to start the regime.

1 How many times a week do you eat yellow, red or orange fruits and vegetables?
- **A** Every day. /
- **B** Most days.
- **C** Hardly ever.

2 How many times a week do you eat dark green leafy vegetables?
- **A** Every day. ι
- **B** Most days.
- **C** Hardly ever.

3 How often do you eat processed foods like pork pies, pasties and salami?
- **A** Never – I love cooking proper meals.
- **B** Rarely – but I do eat them three or four ϡ times a week when I'm busy.
- **C** Most of the time – they're so much easier than having to cook.

4 What type of oil or fat do you use for cooking?
- ƒ **A** Olive oil – the best extra-virgin, organic brand I can afford.
- **B** Sunflower, rapeseed (canola) or other seed oil.

- **C** Butter, lard, hard margarine or anything else that's lurking in the fridge.

5 Do you eat oily fish like salmon, sardines or mackerel?
- **A** Yes, at least once a week – I know it's good for me.
- **B** Occasionally – but I know I should eat more.
- **C** Oily fish? What's that?

6 How much water do you drink a day?
- **A** More than 6 glasses.
- **B** 3–6 glasses.
- **C** 2 or less.

7 How many cups of coffee do you drink each day?
- **A** 3 or less.
- **B** 3–6.
- **C** More than 6.

8 Do you (tick as many as you like)
   Smoke
   ✓Drink more than 14 units (women) or 21 units (men) of alcohol a week

Take sleeping pills/tranquillizers/antidepressants
Use recreational drugs

9 How important is exercise to you?
- **A** Very – I go jogging nearly every day.
- **B** Quite important – I probably do half an hour or so three or four times a week. *(3)*
- **C** Not important at all – I've never been sporty and I don't intend to start now!

10 How often do you make time to thoroughly clean and moisturise your skin?
- **A** Every day. *(1)*
- **B** At least three times a week.
- **C** When I get round to it.

11 Is constipation a problem for you?
- **A** Never.
- **B** Occasionally. *(3)*
- **C** It has been for years

12 Do you suffer with an underactive thyroid?
- **A** No I've never had a problem. *(1)*
- **B** I've had a slight problem but don't take any medication.
- **C** Yes I have to take medication every day.

13 Do you have a skin condition which means you have to use steroid creams?
- **A** No. *(1)*
- **B** Occasionally.
- **C** All the time.

14 Do you take the contraceptive pill or HRT?
- **A** No.
- **B** I used to but I've stopped. *(5)*
- **C** Yes.

15 How stressful do you consider your life/work to be?
- **A** Not very.
- **B** Occasionally when I'm under pressure at home or work.
- **C** Very, all the time. *(5)*

Score: 30
A – 1 point
B – 3 points
C or tick – 5 points

Over 85 – start detoxing now. If you're under 20 you can probably get away with your lifestyle and eating habits but like Dorian Gray, the day will come when everything turns to dust and your radiance will be gone for good. Once you've worked your way through the Radiance Detox, you must then include as many as possible of the protective foods I recommend in your regular diet.

60–85 – all is not lost. A few changes to your eating and lifestyle, a bit more routine skin care and you'll soon be more radiant than ever before. Pay special attention to the Replenishing for Radiance Plan (pages 28–35).

35–60 – you're doing a great job. You're probably eating well, taking care of your skin, enjoying work and home and have very few problems with wrinkles or cellulite.

15–35 – you may be looking great, but I suspect your life is boring. Beauty is more than skin-deep.

cleansing for

Radiance is difficult to measure and even harder to describe, but we all know it when we see it. Bad hair days, lacklustre eyes and sallow skin don't make anyone look very radiant. No detox regime is going to make up for years of smoking, drinking and burning the candle at both ends, so if these habits are the cause of your lack of radiance, they must be tackled now.

But if you're young and willing, you can boost and maintain your natural youthful radiance with appropriate detoxing. Even if you're not so young and the first flush of youth has passed you by, it's not too late. Your skin is a remarkable organ and totally replaces itself with a new layer roughly every six weeks, so you still have a chance to rekindle your radiance.

when should I detox?

Regular twenty-four hour juice fasts are a powerful weapon in the defence of your radiance and even if you have unblemished skin, it's great to follow the twenty-four hour plan at least once a month. Extend it to the forty-eight hour plan in extraordinary situations, for example after indulging in too many Easter eggs, or when you're having an extra stressful time at work. Four times a year, to coincide with the seasons, you should do the full three-day detox as a radiance renewing exercise. It's particularly effective after Christmas and in early spring to make up for over-indulgence, bad weather and lack of sunshine. And if you repeat it in late summer and again in late autumn, it will pump your system full of protective antioxidants that help give you a healthy glow throughout the winter months. If you need to fast for therapeutic reasons, to restore your radiance after illness, injury or periods of severe stress, then the three-day programme is again ideal.

radiance

The twenty-four and forty-eight hour plans are real fasts. The twenty-four hour fast includes no solid food at all, and the forty-eight hour one very little – just some fresh and dried fruit and some nuts. The three-day programme introduces yoghurt, cooked vegetables, a soup and pasta. This fast is certainly not suitable to do while you're working as you need at least one day to recover before going back to your normal activities. For example, start on Friday while you are at work, complete the fast on Saturday and Sunday, then have Monday as a day off.

side effects

You're bound to have some side effects, but don't worry. They're a sign the detox is working.

▶ Headache – this can happen even on a twenty-four hour programme. It's triggered by a drop in your blood-sugar level and the beginnings of elimination, but often it's caused by the body being deprived of caffeine. The more coffee you drink, the worse the headache will pobably be. Don't take painkillers – just drink plenty of water and it will pass.

▶ 'Healing crisis' – increased temperature, sweating, tremors and general aches and pains. Traditionally believed to be caused by the sudden release of accumulated toxins, but now known to be the result of the natural bacteria in the gut dying off and releasing chemicals. These are then absorbed by the gut wall.

cautions

If you suffer with any health problems, always consult your regular physician before starting a detox programme.

the extras

Please don't start any of the plans without being fully prepared. Read through them in detail and make sure you stock up on the foods and supplements that you're going to need as there's nothing more frustrating than getting ready mentally, putting up with the first day and then not being able to complete your detox as effectively as possible.

what to drink

With all my detox programmes I recommend that first thing in the morning you make up a jug of parsley tea from 2 tbsp chopped fresh parsley steeped for 10 minutes in half a litre of boiling water. Strain, cool and keep in the fridge. Drink small glasses regularly throughout the day. This gentle diuretic will help to speed up the detoxifying and cleansing processes, so make sure you drink it all.

Similarly, I always advise that while you can drink as much water, herb or weak China tea as you like, you shouldn't add milk or any sweetening. And you mustn't consume fizzy water, canned drinks, squashes, cordials, alcohol, Indian tea, coffee or any sweetened drinks. This includes sugar-free commercial drinks, which contain artificial sweeteners.

the supplements

As with any detox programme, whether it's the twenty-four-hour detox, the forty-eight-hour detox, the three-day detox, or the eight-day return-to-normal, you can improve the efficiency of the programme and support your body's whole system by using the appropriate supplements every day.

for general well-being

When you're following these programmes, you'll be consuming far less food than normal. Even though the recommended foods provide an abundance of nutrients, it's important to give the body an extra supportive boost of vitamins and minerals to avoid any possible deficiencies and to guarantee optimum levels. For this reason you should take:

▶ 1 high-potency multi-vitamin and mineral supplement (choose one of the reputable brand leaders)

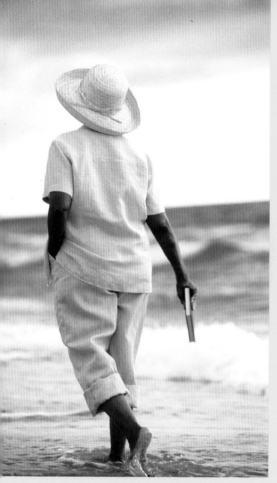

▶ 500 mg vitamin C, three times a day. If you can find it, use ester-C, which many leading manufacturers are now including in their products as it is non-acidic and less likely to cause digestive upsets, especially while you're eating less food

▶ A one-a-day standardized extract of cynarin – from globe artichokes. Cynarin stimulates liver function and helps the body to eliminate the many fat-soluble substances that are stored in the liver.

for bowel function

Maintaining proper and regular bowel function is always important but especially when you are detoxing.

▶ To stimulate, improve and maintain bowel function take 1–2 tablespoons of oatbran or ground psyllium seed every night while you follow the plans and, for best results, start the day before. Both provide water-soluble fibre – better described as smoothage rather than roughage.

for all-round radiance

▶ A supplement of selenium with vitamins A, C and E

▶ A supplement of betacarotene, lutein, zeaxanthine and other carotenoids

▶ A probiotic supplement of gut-friendly bacteria

for specific radiance problems

▶ Ginkgo biloba for thread veins, varicose veins and poor peripheral circulation

▶ Evening primrose oil for dry scaly skin and eczema

▶ Magnesium for nail problems

▶ Silica and saw palmetto for thinning hair

exercise

While you're following the detox programmes, take two or three short walks – not more than 10–15 minutes – each day, whatever the weather. Don't jog, run, go to the gym, dig the garden, spring-clean the house or do strenuous DIY jobs, as over-exertion will drain your energy, produce toxic chemical by-products and inhibit your cleansing regime.

twenty-four hour cleansing

Whether you use this twenty-four-hour Cleansing for Radiance fast as a regular radiance boost or feel you need it because you've just had a weekend of rich food and too much alcohol, you'll find it's really worth the effort – just take a look in the mirror twenty-four hours later to see the difference.

It's a short sharp treatment that anyone can fit into a busy life. You'll be more comfortable if you do it when you're not working, but most people in reasonable health can manage these twenty-four hours without taking time off.

on waking   A large glass of hot water with a thick slice of organic unwaxed lemon

breakfast   A large glass of hot water with a thick slice of organic unwaxed lemon
A glass of Radiant Juice (see recipe, page 82)
A mug of nettle tea

mid-morning   A large glass of hot water with a thick slice of organic unwaxed lemon

lunch   A large glass of Tomato Juice with Garlic and Spring Onions (see recipe, page 81)
A mug of nettle tea

mid-afternoon   A large glass of hot water with a thick slice of organic unwaxed lemon

supper   Mango, Kiwi and Pineapple Juice (see recipe, page 83)
A mug of nettle tea

evening   Carrot and Beetroot Juice (see recipe, page 83)

bedtime   A mug of lime-blossom tea

forty-eight hour cleansing

Start by following the Twenty-Four Hour Cleansing for Radiance plan, then have:

on waking A large glass of hot water with a thick slice of organic unwaxed lemon

breakfast A large glass of hot water with a thick slice of organic unwaxed lemon
A large glass of Radiant Juice (see recipe, page 82)
A mug of nettle tea

mid-morning A large glass of hot water with a thick slice of organic unwaxed lemon

lunch A glass of Radiant Lemonade (see recipe, page 82)
A mug of mint tea

mid-afternoon A large glass of hot water with a thick slice of organic unwaxed lemon

supper A large bowl of fresh fruit salad, to include apple, pear, grapes, mango and some berries
– but no banana
A handful of raisins – chew them very slowly – and a handful of fresh, unsalted
cashew nuts
A mug of mint tea

evening A large glass of hot water with a thick slice of organic unwaxed lemon

bedtime A mug of camomile tea with a teaspoon of organic honey

three-day cleansing

You may already have tried the twenty-four or forty-eight hour fasts and I'm sure you were surprised at how easy they were. Now it's time for you to graduate into the 'grown-ups' league. When you wake up on day four your body will feel lighter, your system cleaner and your eyes and skin will have a sparkle and lustre you haven't seen in ages. You'll also be overflowing with all the protective antioxidants you need and you'll almost certainly have lost over a kilo in weight.

These three days are pretty low in calories, providing around 3,000 altogether when your normal intake should be 2,000 a day for women and 3,000 for men. You'll feel hungry from time to time, but don't spoil it by cheating. To help overcome the hunger pangs take two teaspoons of the Swiss Herbal Tonic BioStrath Elixir, three times a day.

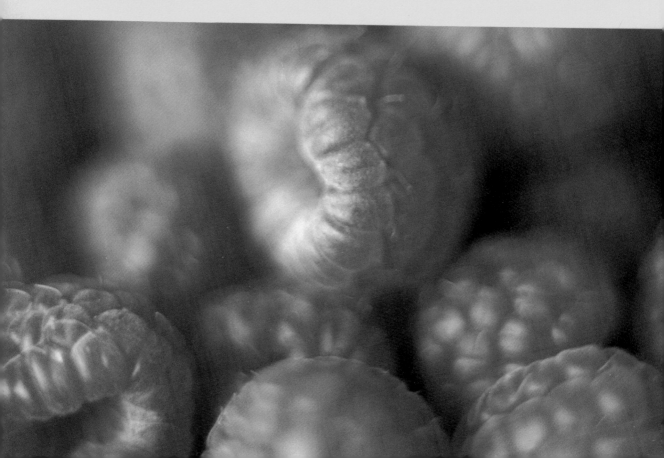

Days 1 and 2, follow the Forty-Eight Hour Cleansing programme. Day 3:

on waking A large glass of hot water with a thick slice of organic unwaxed lemon

breakfast A large glass of hot water with a thick slice of organic unwashed lemon
Fresh fruit salad – a mixture of any of the following: apple, pear, grapes, mango and pineapple and any berries with a carton of live yoghurt and a tablespoon of unsweetened muesli.
A cup of weak Indian tea or herb tea

mid-morning 6 dried apricots
A glass of fruit or vegetable juice

lunch Chilled Watercress Soup (see recipe, page 99) with a chunk of crusty wholemeal bread, no butter
A cup of weak Indian tea or herb tea

mid-afternoon An apple and a pear

supper Courgette Pasta (see recipe, page 89)
A salad of tomato, onion and yellow pepper
A cup of weak Indian tea or herb tea

eight-day return to normal eating

If you're determined to enjoy the long-term radiance benefits which you've already started to build up, then it's really important to go straight on to the return to normal eating programme. Your Radiance Detox has already started the cleansing process, but this is your opportunity to boost your intake of the super-nutrients that your skin, hair and nails require to be in optimum condition. This part of the regime also encourages you into a healthier style of eating which reduces your consumption of the anti-radiance foods, especially those that have a high content of damaging free radicals.

As in all the detox plans, you'll be getting plenty of water to stimulate kidney function and waste elimination – both vital for a clear and radiant skin. The powerful antioxidant dark-coloured berries also feature heavily as they're not only highly protective, but also slow the skin-ageing process and help prevent wrinkles. The plan also gives you lots of vegetable juices rich in the minerals that you need for healthy hair and nails. Probiotic foods like live yoghurt will give you calcium to protect your bones as well as gut-friendly bacteria, which stimulate your immune system and protect against all types of infections, including fungal and bacterial infections of the scalp, nails and skin. You'll also enjoy a wide range of culinary herbs, included for their medicinal value as much as for their flavour. Sage, for example, helps even out hormonal irregularities which can have such a debilitating effect on both skin and hair, and which are often a key factor in the cyclic upsets in your overall radiance.

This is a week of no animal protein and even if you're the most dedicated carnivore, don't cheat. Saturated animal fat is not only a hazard to your heart, blood circulation and blood pressure, it can do severe damage to your radiance. It's a source of free radicals, which attack your body's cells and it can increase the amount of sebum produced by your skin. The result? Your skin will be greasy and more liable to blocked pores and infected spots.

It's important that you follow day 1 exactly as it's laid out here. The following days are more flexible and you may switch light meals and main meals to fit with your lifestyle.

keeping up your fluid intake

As always, you must keep your fluid intake up to a minimum of one and a half litres a day, and avoid canned drinks and commercial juices, just as in the detox plans. Many people find that once they've got into the habit of starting their day with hot water and lemon, it becomes a valuable addition to their normal regime.

Throughout this week take a good quality multivitamin and mineral supplement together with a teaspoon of the Swiss Herbal BioStrath Elixir three times a day.

day 1

This is a very special day when your main food will be rice. Like fasting, rice days are traditionally used by naturopaths as a cleansing treatment. Start by preparing the rice for the whole day. You'll need 100g dry brown rice cooked in half a litre of water. If you prefer, cook half the rice in half the water, and the other half in vegetable stock for a more savoury flavour.

breakfast   85g cooked rice with 140g stewed pears flavoured with honey, cloves and lime juice
A large glass of hot water with a thick slice of organic unwaxed lemon

mid-morning   A large glass of hot water with a thick slice of organic unwaxed lemon

lunch   85g cooked rice with 200g steamed vegetables – celery, thin slices of red and green pepper – tomato purée, garlic and a drizzle of extra-virgin olive oil
A large glass of hot water with a thick slice of organic unwaxed lemon

mid-afternoon   A large glass of hot water with a thick slice of organic unwaxed lemon

supper   85g cooked rice mixed with yoghurt, strawberries, blueberries, banana and kiwi, all whizzed in a blender
A large glass of hot water with a thick slice of organic unwaxed lemon

bedtime   A mug of camomile tea with a teaspoon of organic honey

day 2

breakfast   An orange, half a grapefruit and a large slice of melon
A glass of unsalted vegetable juice, a mug of herb tea

light meal   A plateful of raw red and yellow peppers, cucumber, tomato, broccoli, cauliflower, celery, carrots, radishes and lots of fresh parsley, with extra-virgin olive oil and lemon juice
A large glass of unsweetened fruit juice

main meal   A large salad of lettuce, tomato, watercress, onion, garlic, beetroot, celeriac, fresh mint and any herbs you like, with extra-virgin olive oil and lemon juice
A large glass of unsweetened fruit juice or unsalted vegetable juice

day 3

breakfast   Sliced blood oranges and pink grapefruit
A helping of low-fat live yoghurt, with a teaspoon each of chopped nuts and honey

light meal   Scrambled eggs and mushrooms
Spiced Apricots (make enough for 3 meals) (see recipe, page 103)

main meal   Stuffed Green Peppers (see recipe, page 89)
A large ripe papaya

day 4

breakfast   Spiced Apricots from day 3 with low-fat live yoghurt and an orange

light meal   Potato Cakes with Broccoli (see recipe, page 87)

main meal   Tofu, Vegetable and Cashew Nut Stir-Fry (see recipe, page 90)
Apricot and Almond Crumble (see recipe, page 105)

day 5

breakfast   2 hot wholewheat rolls with a little butter, a banana

light meal   Risotto con Salsa Cruda (see recipe, page 95)

main meal	Aubergine Caviar with Crudités (see recipe, page 100)
	Non-Meatballs in Tomato Sauce (see recipe, page 94)

day 6

breakfast	Spiced Apricots from day 3 with low-fat yoghurt
light meal	Half an avocado, sliced, with watercress, tomatoes and cucumber on mixed leaves with a generous squeeze of lemon juice
	1 crusty wholewheat roll
main meal	Cold Beetroot and Apple Soup (see recipe, page 99)
	Quick Chickpea Casserole (see recipe, page 87)

day 7

breakfast	An orange, apple and a banana
	Low-fat live yoghurt
light meal	Salad Vegeçoise (see recipe, page 101)
main meal	Lentil and Barley Pilaff (see recipe, page 88)
	Pink Grapefruit Sorbet (see recipe, page 103)

day 8

breakfast	A large glass of fresh orange and grapefruit juice
	Cold Spiced Baked Apple (see recipe, page 103) with low-fat live yoghurt, 1 tablespoon oats and three Brazil nuts
light meal	Courgette Pasta (see recipe, page 89)
main meal	Sage Burgers (see recipe, page 92)
	Orange Soufflé Omelette (see recipe, page 102)

cleansing summary

If you've been avoiding mirrors, now's the time to go and take a good look. You may not be quite ready for the illuminated magnifying sort, but you're pretty close. By following this Detox for Cleansing plan, you've done far more than just a favour for your skin – you've cleansed your inner self, and just like an onion, the most important bits are on the inside.

what you've achieved

Even if you've only managed to do a couple of twenty-four hour cleansing fasts you will have already started to regenerate your natural radiance and that should give you the encouragement to be a bit more adventurous. If you've done the three-day detox followed by the eight-day plan, you'll have achieved even more:

- you've helped your body to eliminate a lot of toxic residues
- you've significantly reduced the amount of irritant waste being excreted through your skin
- you've made your liver work more efficiently and drastically lightened its load so that it can start getting rid of the toxic chemicals stored in its fat deposits
- you've stimulated all of your body's natural eliminating processes
- you've improved your digestive function so your body can absorb more of the essential nutrients from the food you eat.

how you feel

One of the most difficult challenges for anyone is to totally change their eating habits. It's hard to give up things you like, but it can be even more difficult to make yourself eat foods which are not a normal part of your daily menus. But over the years I've found that many of my patients who reluctantly embark on these detox programmes feel so much better afterwards and enjoy the food to such an extent, that many of the recipes soon become firm favourites. You'll soon find out why:

▶ Just looking in the mirror will confirm how worthwhile your effort has been – your skin will look clear and radiant and your eyes will be brighter than they've been for ages.

▶ When you brush your hair it will have new lustre and body. Even though the hair you see is mostly dead tissue, a better diet means less grease which attracts less dirt and leaves your hair looking and feeling more natural.

▶ The obvious improvements in your appearance will give you a renewed self-confidence which in turn leads to inner radiance. This will affect the way you move, think and feel.

▶ You may find it hard to believe before you start, but the Super-Radiance Detox will even change the way you dress. You'll be more confident in your choice of colour and style and will no longer settle for wearing drab colours that blend in with the wallpaper.

▶ The most convincing thing of all will be when your family, friends and colleagues comment on the changes they see. They'll probably think you've at least been on holiday and that you've probably had botox treatment, collagen injections or a face lift. Let them think what they like. You'll know the secret of the radiance detox.

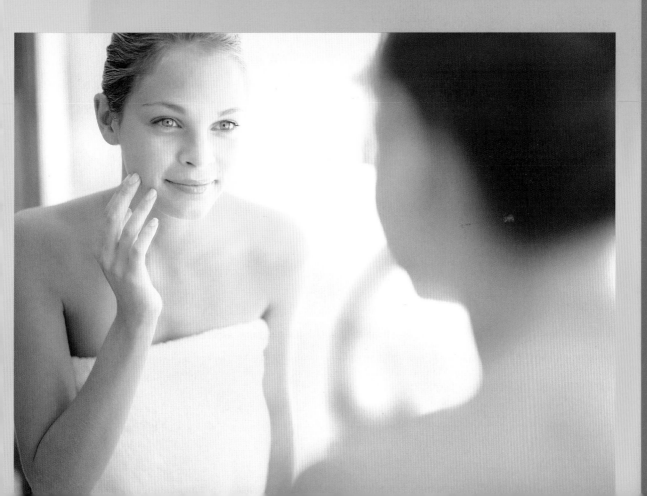

replenishing

Nutritionists have a disconcerting habit of talking about nutrients – vitamins, minerals, calories, carbohydrates, proteins, and so on. Unfortunately real people don't eat nutrients – they eat food. But it's knowing what nutrient-containing foods to eat that's important when it comes to replenishing your lost radiance. As well as vitamins **A** and **E** and zinc, which I've already mentioned on page 9, these are the most important nutrients, why you need them and where to get them. To make sure you replenish and maintain your radiance eat a good selection from all these foods on a very regular basis.

B vitamins

These are essential, especially for the nervous system, while vitamin **B12** also prevents pernicious anaemia. The B vitamins are found in yeast, wholegrain cereals, liver and all meat, and B12 is also in eggs, cheese, yoghurt, yeast extracts and beer. Two teaspoons of liver contain more than a day's B vitamins requirement.

folic acid

This is a vital B vitamin that prevents birth defects and heart disease. It's in vegetables and cereals. Meet your daily needs with 100g of spinach, or 170g of either potatoes, Brussels sprouts, chickpeas, broccoli, kale or asparagus.

vitamin D

This is essential for bone strength, and oily fish, margarine and eggs are the most important sources – 40g of herring or kipper, 60g of mackerel, 85g of tinned salmon or 140g of tinned sardines will all provide your daily requirement.

for radiance

calcium

This is essential for bones. Find virtually all you need in 10g of whitebait, 10g of cheese, 10g of tinned sardines, half a litre of milk (skimmed, semi-skimmed or whole), or 40g of tofu.

magnesium

This is essential for every cell and is important to the way calcium and potassium are utilized by your body. You'll find it in cereals, nuts, green vegetables, beans, peas, millet and in wholemeal bread.

iron

This is vital for blood and the best sources are meat and offal, though whitebait, mussels, cockles and winkles also contain large amounts. Vegetable sources are not so easily absorbed. Get more than your daily dose from 60g of cockles, 140g of liver or 170g of mussels. You can also get valuable amounts of iron from a portion of dahl, a portion of vegetable curry, a portion of beans or a portion of dark-green vegetables.

potassium

This is needed by every cell but isn't stored by the body. Ensure you get enough by making soups or gravies with the water you've cooked your vegetables in. A large baked potato, a portion of vegetable curry, a dozen dried apricots, a herring or a mackerel, a couple of bananas, a watercress salad or a handful of raisins, will make up for any deficiencies.

seven-day replenishing

This is a varied week of super-radiant eating during which you'll be making up for all those skin-nourishing and skin- and body-protective nutrients that have not been part of your regular eating in the past.

You can swap whole days around and you can eat light or main meals in whichever order suits your own personal lifestyle, but you must not mix meals from different days.

And during this week, don't drink more than two cups of coffee or Indian tea a day – that includes decaffeinated versions – but you do need a minimum of one and a half litres of fluid, one litre of which should be water. The rest can be herb or China tea without milk or sugar.

breakfast rules

Every morning this week you should eat the same breakfast, and there are no excuses for not eating it. It is a major part of your radiance programme. If you can find time to get your hair done, fix your make-up, paint your nails, get a tattoo, have your legs waxed or go to therapy, you can find time for breakfast.

The daily standard breakfast to be eaten every day consists of:

▶ A large glass of hot water with a thick slice of unwaxed lemon
▶ A glass of any fresh unsweetened fruit juice or unsalted vegetable juice
▶ A portion of any unsweetened wholegrain breakfast cereal, muesli or porridge with soya milk, 4 prunes and a sprinkling of raisins **or**
▶ A large glass of soya milk whizzed in a blender with a tablespoon of unsalted shelled nuts, 2 dried apricots and a banana

You may also have a cup of tea or coffee.

added extras

Replenishing for Radiance means taking some essential anti-ageing skin-, hair- and nail-nourishing nutrients every day. You should stick to this group of supplements for up to six weeks, after which you shouldn't need them unless you have specific health concerns like anaemia or menopausal problems, or if you are on long-term medication. In these cases it is beneficial to carry on for longer:

▶ A plant-hormone extract from either soya or red clover
▶ 200 International Units of vitamin E
▶ 1 one-a-day multi-mineral supplement which includes calcium, potassium, selenium, boron, iodine and zinc
▶ An antioxidant, vitamin and carotenoid supplement that includes vitamins A, C, E, B6, B12 and folic acid
▶ 500mg evening primrose oil

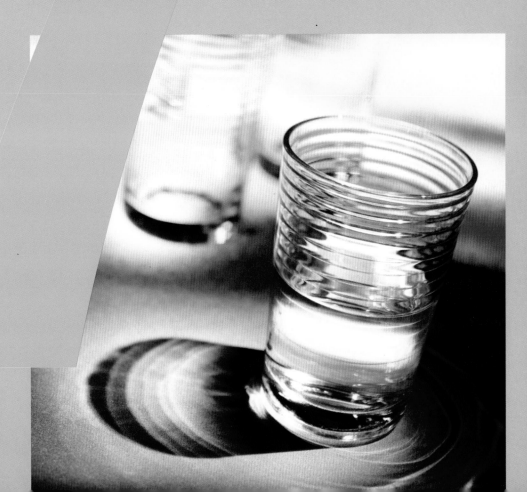

day 1

light meal   Tomato Risotto (see recipe, page 89) with a salad of chicory, cucumber, carrot and celery
A thick slice of cantaloupe melon

main meal   Grilled Sole with Cheese (see recipe, page 87) with steamed broccoli, mange tout and
sweetcorn served with olive oil and lemon and sprinkled with toasted pumpkin seeds
A large pear

day 2

light meal   Pasta with Tuna Fish and Black Olives (see recipe, page 90)
Mixed salad with oil-and-vinegar dressing, sprinkled with toasted sunflower seeds
Kiwi and Passion Fruit Smoothie (see recipe, page 83), replacing the milk with soya milk

main meal   Chicken Liver Kebabs (see recipe, page 88) with wholemeal pitta
A large salad of lettuce, rocket, watercress, parsley and mint with an olive-oil and lemon-
juice dressing
Soya Blueberry and Strawberry Smoothie (see recipe, page 82)

day 3

light meal   Pitta-Bread Pizza (see recipe, page 95) with a large bowl of Crudités with Garlic
Mayonnaise (see recipe, page 101)
Mixture of dried ready-to-eat apricots, dates and walnuts

main meal   Bean Casserole (see recipe, page 91)
Salad of sliced radishes, spring onions, lamb's lettuce, rocket and parsley
Spiced Baked Apple (see recipe, page 103)

day 4

light meal   Scrambled Eggs with Smoked Mackerel (see recipe, page 91) and wholemeal toast
Sliced avocado and tomato salad sprinkled with toasted sunflower and pumpkin seeds
Fruit salad made from fresh grapefruit and orange with lime juice

main meal   Grilled Paprika Chicken (see recipe, page 95) with new potatoes, pak choi and French
beans sprinkled with chopped garlic and a drizzle of olive oil and lemon juice
Fresh Fruit Brûlée (see recipe, page 102)

day 5

light meal   Pasta with Tuna Fish and Black Olives (see recipe, page 90)
Salad of watercress, beansprout, chicory and mushrooms
2 kiwi fruit

main meal   Stir-Fried Turkey Breast with Vegetables and Noodles (see recipe, page 85)
Carrot and Melon Salad (see recipe, page 101)
Spiced Apricots (see recipe, page 103)

day 6

light meal   Chilled Avocado Soup (see recipe, page 98)
Rye crispbread with your favourite cheese
Mango and Soya Milk Smoothie (see recipe, page 83)

main meal   Baked Halibut with Mushrooms (see recipe, page 94) served with brown rice and mixed
stir-fried vegetables
Apricot and Almond Crumble (see recipe, page 105)

day 7

light meal   Potato Cakes with Broccoli (see recipe, page 87) with chicory, cucumber, carrot and
celery salad
A small bunch of red grapes

main meal   Chicken with Thyme and Lemon (see recipe, page 94) with boiled rice and Ratatouille
(see recipe, page 85)
Stewed Pears with Mascarpone and Cloves (see recipe, page 102)

replenishing summary

After this past seven days of Replenishing for Radiance, you've had another week without consuming any high-fat, high-sugar or high-salt convenience and ready-made foods, so you've made a major breakthrough as far as improving and maintaining your natural radiance is concerned.

what you've achieved

The replenishing programme you've just followed has been high in antioxidants and rich in super-radiance nutrients, but hasn't had all those E-numbers, preservatives or chemical additives that add to the toxic load of your body. It has also spared you the 12g of salt that the average person consumes each day — the safe maximum is 5g. As a result of all this you've achieved:

▶ A considerable reduction in the amount of fluid your body is retaining
▶ A significant boost to the levels of skin-protective antioxidants circulating in your blood
▶ Unless you've cheated, you haven't introduced any toxic chemicals into your body
▶ You have increased the quantity of cell-nourishing and building nutrients in your body
▶ You have ensured that your skin, hair and nails have all the nutrients they need for repair and replacement
▶ You have guaranteed optimum protection for your bones.

how you feel

You are entitled to feel just a bit like the cat who's got the cream — and you'll get some of that in a fortnight as no real food is forbidden in the radiance programme. You'll have a new spring in your step and a growing awareness of the truth in the old proverb 'you are what you eat'.

▶ You are enjoying a new sense of self-esteem and as well as fulfilling all your other commitments, you've taken time and effort to care for yourself.

▶ You are feeling more confident every day about the appearance you present to the outside world.

▶ You'll feel surprised because, despite the fact that you have probably eaten considerably more than normal, you've lost a kilo or so in weight. Those slightly tight jeans will be a bit baggy, the posh frock that strained a little across the waist will be comfortable, and you'll even find some outfits you haven't worn for years that make you look terrific.

▶ You'll feel more secure in your relationships as you develop a growing sense of satisfaction with yourself.

▶ You may feel just a little discouraged because you won't, at this stage, see the same dramatic changes as after the initial Cleansing for Radiance detox programme. But be patient. Over the next few weeks you'll blossom into full bloom.

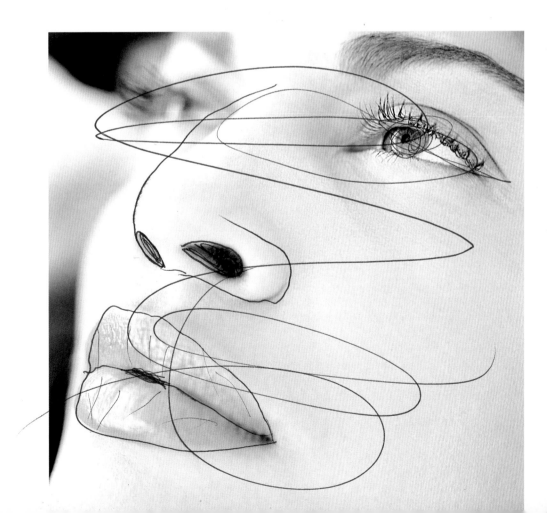

rebuilding for

Now's the time to think about rebuilding your lifestyle and eating for permanent and easily maintained radiance. Having got this far you really have already made a major impact on your body's ability to protect and maintain all the visible aspects of your radiance – a healthy skin, lustrous hair and strong, beautiful nails. This is not the time to throw all these hard-won gains away. After all, it hasn't been easy and to follow the plans this far has required a great deal of effort, organization and self-discipline.

If you follow the Rebuilding for Radiance programme, I know from my own patients that most of you will end up incorporating the basic concepts into your everyday living on a permanent basis. Equally important is the fact that if you are also shopping and cooking for a family, the overall health benefits as well as the radiance-boosting effects will be passed on to the others, and particularly to your children, and will become part of their normal eating habits, too.

This Rebuilding programme should be followed exactly as set out the first time you do it so that you get a feel for the type of foods which are essential at this stage. However, once you've got the hang of it, you will easily work out substitute ingredients and will incorporate favourite recipes that will provide the same radiance-boosting benefits but that may fit more comfortably with your own particular likes and dislikes and the lifestyle of you and your family.

The whole object of Rebuilding for Radiance is to provide you with the tools you need to eat abundantly of radiance-boosting foods with the minimum of effort and in such a way that you

radiance

hardly have to think about it because it has become a daily routine. Instead of reaching for the instant noodles or microwaveable ready-meal, you automatically choose fresh pasta, nuts and seeds for skin-nourishing minerals, dark-green leafy vegetables for their anti-bacterial and skin-protective sulphur compounds, dried fruits for their beta-carotene, which is vital for the growth of new skin cells, and soya products for their plant hormones that take care of your hair and skin.

One of the biggest problems I have with my own patients is their sometimes strange and inappropriate concept of what is healthy. Thanks to the lunatic fringe of bogus nutritionists, vast numbers of women have stopped eating a wide range of foods in the belief that they are either fattening or unhealthy, and this includes some of the most important radiance-boosting foods. Something like 30 per cent of women believe they're allergic to wheat and dairy products, while in reality less than 2 per cent of the population has allergies to these foods. Sadly for these women, both these food groups contain nutrients which hold the key to healthy skin, hair and nails. Similarly, women don't eat avocados, one of the richest sources of vitamin E, another essential skin and hair nutrient. Many women also avoid eggs because of their cholesterol content, but this is yet another of those nutritional myths. Eggs are, in fact, an excellent source of iron, B vitamins and lecithin – all super-radiance nutrients for skin, hair and nails.

As I've said before, to rebuild your radiance the simple answer is a diet that combines the widest possible range of different foods. Only this is your guarantee of an optimum intake of radiant nutrients.

fourteen-day rebuilding

This fourteen-day Rebuilding for Radiance regime starts by repeating the seven-day Replenishing for Radiance plan. I'm sure you'll agree that the food was varied and interesting, as well as tasting good. The recipes in it are all extremely healthy and not at all cranky. That makes them perfect for everyone in the family, so you won't have to be cooking two lots of meals all the time.

When it comes to the Rebuilding regime, breakfasts loom large again and it really is vital that you eat one of the alternatives every single day. They provide the phytoestrogens that help balance your hormone levels and they are a rich source of B vitamins, fibre and minerals. On top of that, they give you a combination of instant- and slow-release energy. This is what perks you up in the morning and keeps you going till lunch time so you don't have that mid-morning sugar craving that leads to radiance-destroying unhealthy snacks.

During this week do not drink more than four cups of coffee or Indian tea a day – that includes decaffeinated versions – but you need a minimum of one and a half litres of fluid, one litre of which should be water. The rest can be herb or China tea without milk or sugar.

You can switch the meals around on each day and can switch whole days, but don't take breakfast from one day, a light meal from another and a main meal from a third, as this won't give you the daily balance you need.

You should still be taking your Replenishing for Radiance extras and should continue with them throughout this Rebuilding regime. Here are your menus for week two.

Days 1–7, follow the Seven-Day Replenishing programme.

day 8

breakfast A glass of fresh unsweetened fruit juice or unsalted vegetable juice

2 poached eggs and one poached tomato on an unbuttered slice of wholemeal bread (toasted or untoasted)

light meal Tomato Risotto (see recipe, page 89) with a salad of chicory, cucumber, carrot and celery

A thick slice of Radiance Teabread (see recipe, page 79)

main meal Salmon Fishcakes with Tomato Salsa (see recipe, page 86), with steamed Chinese cabbage, courgettes and new potatoes in their skins

Stewed Pears with Mascarpone and Cloves (see recipe, page 102)

day 9

breakfast A glass of fresh unsweetened fruit juice or unsalted vegetable juice

A large helping of fresh blueberries, raspberries, currants, strawberries – whatever is in season – with a carton of live natural yoghurt, sprinkled with 1 dessertspoon of wheatgerm and 1 dessertspoon of toasted linseeds

light meal Aubergine Caviar with Crudités (see recipe, page 100) with warm wholemeal pitta bread

Fresh fruit salad

main meal Prawn and Tomato Curry (see recipe, page 84) with brown rice and mixed green salad

A bowl of live natural yoghurt sprinkled with toasted almonds and a drizzle of honey

day 10

breakfast A glass of fresh unsweetened fruit juice or unsalted vegetable juice

1 fresh peach sliced into a bowl of organic low-salt wholewheat flakes, with chilled soya milk and 1 dessertspoon of flaked almonds

light meal 1 sliced avocado with Broad Bean, Tomato and Herb Salad (see recipe, page 100), with 2 rice cakes

Pink Grapefruit Sorbet (see recipe, page 103)

main meal   Sweetcorn and Haddock Chowder (see recipe, page 98)

A good chunk of My Easy Bread (see recipe, page 78)

A green leaf salad with fresh chopped mint, thyme and dill, and a squeeze of lemon juice

A small piece of goat's cheese and a fresh peach

day 11

breakfast   Fresh strawberry and banana smoothie made with half live natural yoghurt and
half soya milk

1 slice of wholemeal bread or toast with a thin slice of Dutch cheese

light meal   A fruit cocktail made of fresh orange, kiwi and grapefruit

Eggs Florentine (see recipe, page 86) with fingers of wholemeal toast

Buckwheat Crêpes (see recipe, page 104), sprinkled with raisins and replacing the honey
with maple syrup

main meal   Spinach Soup with Yoghurt (see recipe, page 99)

Quick Chickpea Casserole (see recipe, page 87)

Salad of large plum, cherry and sun-dried tomatoes sprinkled with torn basil and
drizzled with olive oil

Any seasonal fresh fruit

day 12

breakfast   A glass of fresh unsweetened fruit juice or unsalted vegetable juice

A large bowl of fresh chopped apple, pear, kiwi, mango and papaya with a generous
squeeze of lime juice

1 slice of wholemeal toast with a little butter and organic honey

light meal   Watercress Soup (see recipe, page 99)

Dark rye bread with a generous portion of your favourite cheeses and an apple
and a few grapes

main meal   Griddled Tuna with Roasted Vegetables and Fusilli (see recipe, page 92)

Fresh Cherry Tart (see recipe, page 105)

day 13

breakfast A glass of fresh unsweetened fruit juice or unsalted vegetable juice

Colcannon (see recipe, page 80)

light meal A large Greek Salad (see recipe, page 100) with warm wholemeal pitta bread

Yoghurt, Papaya and Kiwi Smoothie (see recipe, page 83)

main meal Salad of baby artichoke hearts, peas, carrots and mint with olive oil and cider-vinegar dressing

Chicken Liver Kebabs (see recipe, page 88) on a bed of rice

Any stewed fruit with live yoghurt

day 14

breakfast A glass of fresh unsweetened fruit juice or unsalted vegetable juice

Half a pink grapefruit

Cinnamon Toast with Figs (see recipe, page 79)

light meal One-Pot Pasta with Vegetables and Pesto (see recipe, page 93)

Half an ogen melon filled with mixed berries

main meal Potted Shrimps (see recipe, page 84)

Beef and Ginger Stir-Fry (see recipe, page 93)

A bowl of soaked dried fruits

rebuilding summary

Now you're positively glowing. If you've done things according to the plan, you've had three consecutive weeks of a dietary regime that simply oozes the nutrients your body needs to rebuild your radiance. Every day you've lost millions of dead skin cells and the last three weeks have provided you with the essentials you need to start to replace them with the healthiest possible cells. Remember, it takes the body at least six weeks to cover itself with a completely new outer layer of skin.

What's more, now that your other eliminating processes are working more efficiently and your diet doesn't contain the body pollutants that it used to, you're producing less waste for the skin to excrete, and that must be good because that waste is a skin irritant.

what you've achieved

▶ By boosting your consumption of all the key nutrients, your blood is now able to take better care of your skin. The tiniest blood vessels are carrying optimum amounts of protein, essential fatty acids, minerals, vitamins, energy and oxygen to every skin cell.

▶ The B vitamins you've consumed are nourishing your whole nervous system, including the millions of tiny nerve-endings that control the skin's activities.

▶ Your nails and hair are in good condition now thanks to these same nutrients and thanks to the zinc and calcium boost you've had.

▶ Your hair is particularly revitalised. There's an improvement in the new hair growing out of each hair follicle, though you may not see the improvement yet.

▶ Your eyes will be at their brightest as you've consumed exceptionally high levels of the eye-protective carotenoids in recent weeks. These nutrients also offer enormous long-term protection against cataracts and age-related macular degeneration.

how you feel

▶ You feel attractive and that makes you feel good inside. This has nothing to do with height, size, weight, skin colour or preconceptions of beauty. It's all about knowing you're doing the best you can and feeling that you've made the effort.

▶ Your skin feels softer, smoother and much more supple.

▶ You feel happy because your hair is more manageable and your nails are finally growing and getting less brittle.

▶ You have a feeling of energy and enthusiasm that goes hand in hand with your increased store of radiance.

▶ You feel determined that you're never going back to your old habits – all that junk food, those endless cups of coffee at your desk and the lack of time to take care of yourself. This is very definitely the new you.

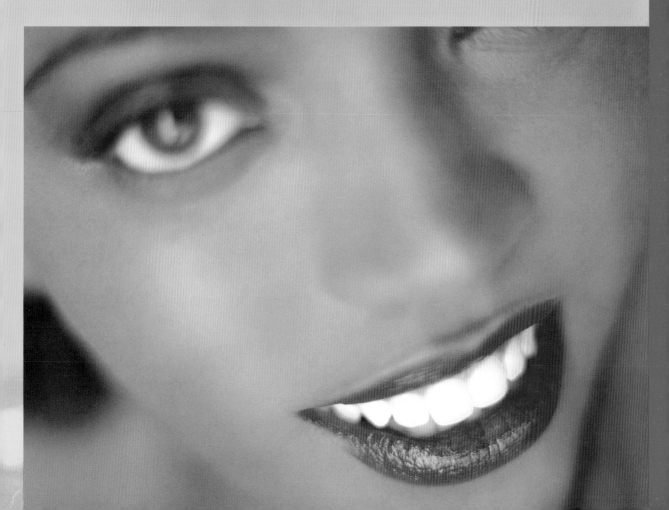

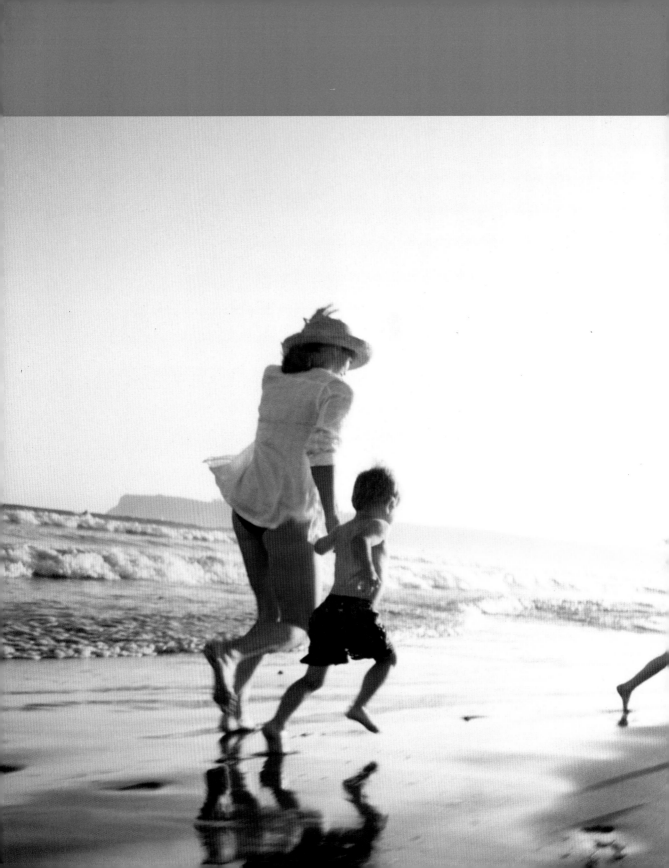

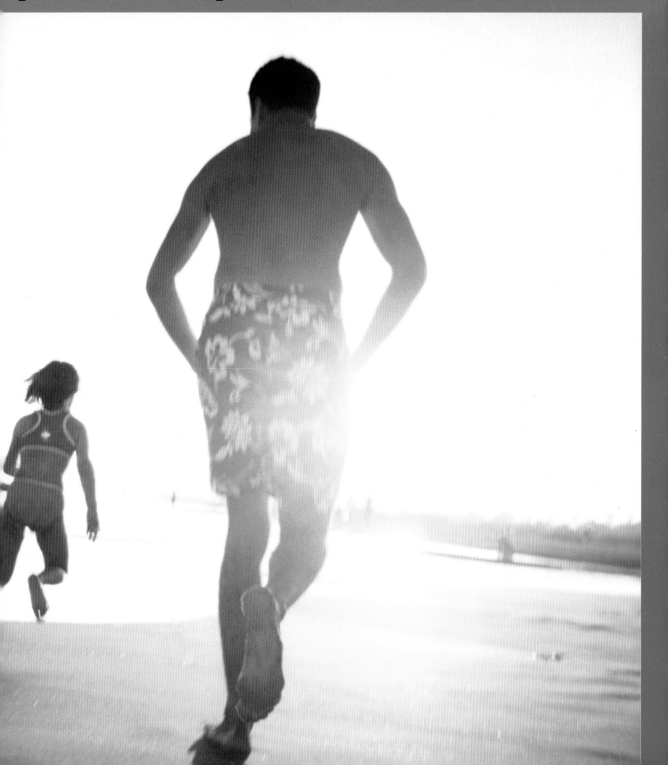

part 2 super radiance for life

radiant minds for

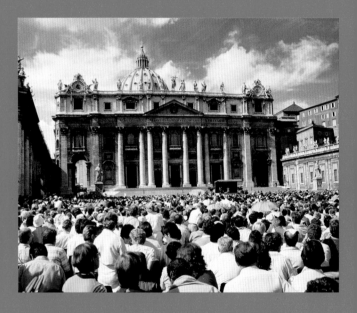

Radiance stems from both the physical and the spiritual. You won't have perfect hair, skin and nails if your body is deficient in essential nutrients or awash with toxic pollutants from food, drink or the environment. But radiance is multi-factorial and while good nutrition will give you a sound foundation, there are physical and emotional factors which can have a powerful influence – positive or negative – on your radiant state.

On the emotional side, everyone has to deal with negative emotions such as stress, depression, anger, hate, spite and jealousy. So that these emotions don't destroy your radiance, you need to learn how to deal with them. Take stress, for example. Not all stress is bad and in fact, you can learn how to use well-controlled stress to your advantage. And when stress does strike, follow my simple tips for keeping it to a minimum. You'll see just how well you can survive and keep your radiance intact.

On the physical side, age-old therapies such as massage and aromatherapy can give a huge boost to your overall feelings of well-being, and these will complement the nutritional radiance benefits gained from your already improved diet. Part of the radiance benefits of massage come from the healing power of touch, regardless of the type of massage, but the benefits

radiant bodies

don't come only from a professional massage. In fact, there's no reason why anyone shouldn't give a massage to a friend or partner as, with very few exceptions, it's impossible to do any harm. And perhaps the most surprising fact is that the giver derives almost as much radiance-boosting benefit as the receiver. I know. I've been doing it for 40 years. Just try for yourself.

Another facet to the physical side of radiance, is physical activity. Few people associate this with radiance, but without a shadow of doubt, taking regular exercise benefits your overall well-being, your heart and circulation and consequently your skin and hair. In terms of your overall well-being, it generates the release of the brain's own feel-good chemicals – endorphins – so after exercise you won't just glow from exertion, but also from happy, radiant feelings. Physical activity will also increase the amount of oxygen in your blood and will stimulate your heart rate and the amount of blood pumped through your system. This in turn will carry more nutrients to your skin and hair follicles, and the result will be healthier and more radiant skin and hair. But whatever you do, don't be tempted to become a marathon runner or an obsessive exerciser as doing this will have a serious negative impact on your radiance and general health. Modest exercise three or four times a week is all you need.

And last but not least comes radiance-boosting laughter. Although you may think it sounds like an old wives' tale, laughter really is the best medicine, and there's now a lot of scientific evidence to prove it. But you don't need me to tell you that watching somebody who is smiling and laughing is a much more radiant vision than sitting opposite someone at dinner whose mouth is permanently turned down and whose brow is furrowed in a frown.

beat the stress

Some stress is essential to normal life and it's often the adrenaline generated by stress that powers creativity. The problems occur when stress becomes relentless and excessive. Apart from the repercussions on your health – high blood pressure, strokes, heart disease, anxiety, insomnia and a host of other medical problems – nothing affects your radiance to the same degree. Your posture suffers and you droop. The blood supply to your skin is diminished, and you look grey and puffy. Constant tension and anxiety lead to headaches, which result in frowning and worry lines. None of this make you feel or look your radiant best.

You may not realise how much stress you're under so how do you tell whether you are suffering from too much? Check the questionnaire below and see how you score. Do you:

▶ feel near to tears much of the time?

▶ fidget, bite your nails or fiddle with your hair?

▶ find it hard to concentrate, and impossible to make decisions?

▶ find it increasingly hard to talk to people?

▶ snap and shout at those around you at home and work?

▶ eat when you're not hungry?

▶ feel tired much of the time?

▶ think that your sense of humour has gone for good?

▶ feel suspicious of others?

▶ no longer have any interest in sex?

▶ sleep badly?

▶ drink and/or smoke more to help you through those difficult days?

▶ ever feel that you just can't cope?

If you answer **yes** to more than four of these questions, you are stressed. **Do something!** You can't carry on this way.

de-stress the distress

Here's how to break out of the cycle.

▶ Do not work more than nine hours a day.

▶ Take at least half an hour off in the day.

▶ Take at least one and a half days out of your normal working routine each week.

▶ Eat regular and healthy meals.

▶ Take regular exercise.

▶ Practise some form of relaxation technique.

▶ Do not use alcohol, caffeine, nicotine, or drugs to relieve stress.

▶ Remember that stressful situations are not always the unhappy ones. Getting married, promoted or moving house all cause stress.

▶ Learn to recognise your own stress thresholds.

▶ Use stress positively and channel your energy into making your life better.

blissful massage

A good massage is relaxing, luxurious, pampering and extremely therapeutic. It induces feelings of inner calm, peace and well-being, relaxes tense muscles, soothes away headaches and other aches and pains, and relieves physical and emotional tension. It shouldn't be seen as self-indulgence but as an important part of your detoxing for radiance programme. And apart from all these wonderful benefits, massage can stimulate the lymph drainage system and speed up the body's eliminating processes.

The effects of massage are cumulative and when used regularly, its benefits soon become apparent. Many of my patients have regular massages and a number of them now suffer far less from distress, anxiety, depression, migraine and even high blood pressure. Some can now even do without medication, though it goes without saying that you must never

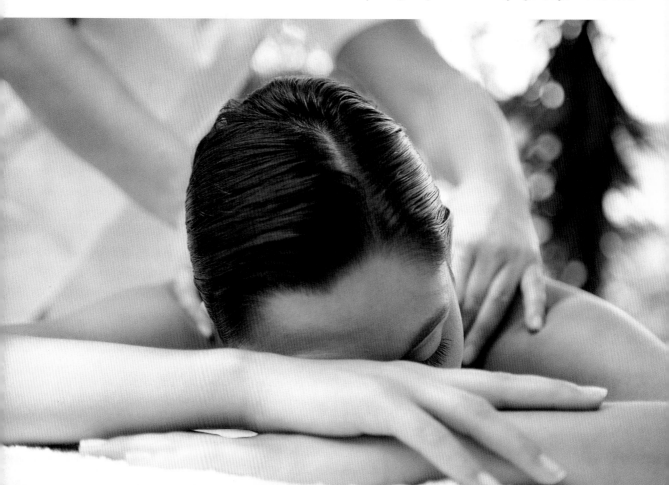

change or stop any prescribed long-term medication without the co-operation and approval of your own professional health adviser.

take care

Do not have a massage if you suffer from any of the following:

▶ Thrombosis, phlebitis or cellulitis

▶ Leg ulcers

▶ Inflamed joints after injury or acute arthritis

▶ High temperature

▶ Varicose veins

▶ Unexplained large bruises

▶ Any skin condition which is obviously infected, weeping or suppurating.

giving a massage

When giving a massage, use rhythmic, repetitive movements and avoid pressing down on bony areas as this would be uncomfortable. Many people find it a good idea to play their favourite slow music in the background so they can work in time with the rhythm. Western massage is based on four separate techniques which can be used separately or in any combination.

▶ Effleurage is a rhythmic stroking movement that produces physical and mental relaxation. Effleurage movements are made towards the heart.

▶ Petrissage is a bit like kneading bread dough. It's a deep lifting, rolling and squeezing movement, which stimulates muscles and fatty tissue. It's valuable as a way of stretching and relaxing contracted muscles.

▶ Pressure is applied using small rotating movements of the thumbs, fingertips or heel of the hand. It's used in small specific areas of tension in the neck, shoulders and buttocks. If you're a small person dealing with a large body you can sometimes get more pressure by using the point of your elbow.

▶ Percussion is a really hard technique for an amateur to master as it uses fast rhythmic slaps with either a cupped hand or the little finger edge of the hand. It can be used to stimulate skin, blood flow and breathing.

the ancient art of aromatherapy

You may think aromatherapy is yet another 'new age' gimmick, but you'd be wrong. The use of essential oils is at least three thousand years old. From the Aztecs to the ancient Greeks and from the Romans to the early Christian church, the mood-enhancing and medicinal properties of these oils have long been recognized.

There are various ways of enjoying essential oils. You can burn them in a fragrancer so you breathe in their volatile vapours, or you can use them as an inhalation. Add three drops to a large bowl of hot water, cover your head and the bowl with a towel, keep your eyes closed and breathe in through the nose and out through the mouth for three or four minutes.

To use essential oils for skin massage, dilute them with a vegetable carrier oil like grapeseed, sunflower, corn or almond oil and then apply. When making up mixtures for massage oil don't use more than two drops of essential oil to each large teaspoon of carrier.

You can even add a few drops to your bathwater, but steer well clear of thyme, basil, clove, cinnamon or peppermint oil as these may irritate the skin. And be sure to avoid direct application of all essential oils during pregnancy without professional advice, as some oils could be harmful.

good-mood mixes

Different oils have different effects on your mood, but whichever you choose, you'll achieve a more radiant mind which, in turn, will help you towards a more radiant body. Here are some of the most effective good-mood oil mixes around. For the massage oils, dilute the total number of total drops with one tablespoon of carrier oil.

vitality

massage – 3 drops lemon, 2 drops geranium, 1 drop frankincense
fragrancer – bergamot
bath – grapefruit

brain

massage – 2 drops rosemary, 3 drops thyme, 1 drop basil
fragrancer – lemon grass
bath – fennel and juniper

snooze

massage – 3 drops neroli, 3 drops geranium, 2 drops lavender
fragrancer – lavender
bath – mimosa

wake up

massage – 2 drops pine, 4 drops juniper
fragrancer – eucalyptus and lime
bath – juniper

sexy

massage – 4 drops rose otto, 2 drops jasmine, 2 drops sandalwood
fragrancer – sandalwood
bath – ylang ylang

macho

massage – 3 drops cedarwood, 2 drops thyme, 2 drops cypress
fragrancer – sandalwood and cinnamon
bath – patchouli

sensitive

massage – 2 drops jasmine, 2 drops lime blossom, 2 drops neroli, 1 drop carnation
fragrancer – jasmine and carnation
bath – hyacinth

get rid of your anger

Just like excessive stress, anger causes resentment, bitterness and anxiety. If you let it get the better of you, it not only damages your health, but has a powerful negative effect on how radiant you look and feel. Not surprisingly, the trick is to learn to let your anger out.

Attitudes to letting go of your anger vary enormously in different parts of the world. For example, the Anglo-Saxon approach is very different to the Mediterranean one. If you're Anglo-Saxon, it's not done to lose your temper, but watch an Italian, Spanish or Greek family eating Sunday lunch and from all the shouting and gesticulating, you'd imagine they were in the middle of a 50-year feud. In reality, they're probably only arguing about whether there's too much salt in the soup.

People from the Mediterranean have no inhibitions about showing their anger and I'm sure this is why in the Mediterranean, even great-grandmothers, weather-beaten and wrinkled though they may be, exude boundless radiance.

how to let go

There are many ways to release the pent-up anger and frustrations of day-to-day living and it's far safer to do so in a controlled and purposeful way than to let the pressure build and build until you finally get sick or explode into a violent rage.

Physical exercise is especially recommended by the experts. It gets rid of excess energy, encourages self-confidence and offers a safe environment for you to use your anger in a competitive way. It's known, for example, that endurance runners, who run long distances each week, tend to be less anxious, more emotionally stable and less prone to irrational outbursts of anger than their physically less active contemporaries.

If sport's not your thing, find out what works for you. For some, it's a hobby like gardening or painting; for others, the cinema, theatre or music.

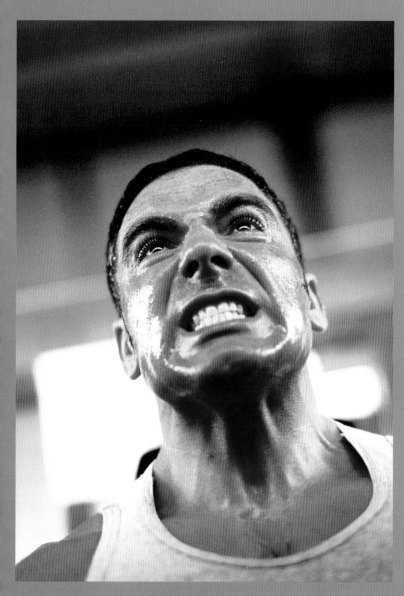

I was once at the Tivoli Gardens in Copenhagen where the local pottery had a stand full of their seconds. For just a small cost, you could hurl a pile of reject plates at a brick wall. It was a perfect way to get rid of any anger. If you don't happen to have a handy store of old china, try hanging a rug in the garden and beating it with a tennis racket, or having a punch bag in your bedroom. Then, after a frustrating day when the boss has been on your back or you've been given a parking ticket, you can have a five-minute workout. Hit and punch away, shout and scream, just lose your inhibitions. You'll be amazed at how relaxed and calm you feel afterwards. It's all too easy to criticise people who have a short fuse, but unless their anger turns to violence, they are better off than people who, as a result of years of conditioning, find it impossible to show any anger or annoyance.

If you're in any doubt, just think of the fun you had last time you smashed some plates at a Greek taverna!

smile and the world smiles with you

To boost your radiance even more, you must remember to smile. It requires much more effort to frown than to smile as frowning uses many more muscles. And it's frowning that leaves you with a wrinkled forehead, droopy skin at the corners of your eyes and a miserable down-turned mouth. Smiling on the other hand makes you feel good and look radiant. And surprising though it may seem, smiling brings skin-protective benefits. There's now a mass of scientific evidence proving conclusively that positive attitudes enhance the body's immune defences and so protect your skin – and all your other organs too – from the ageing damage of free radicals.

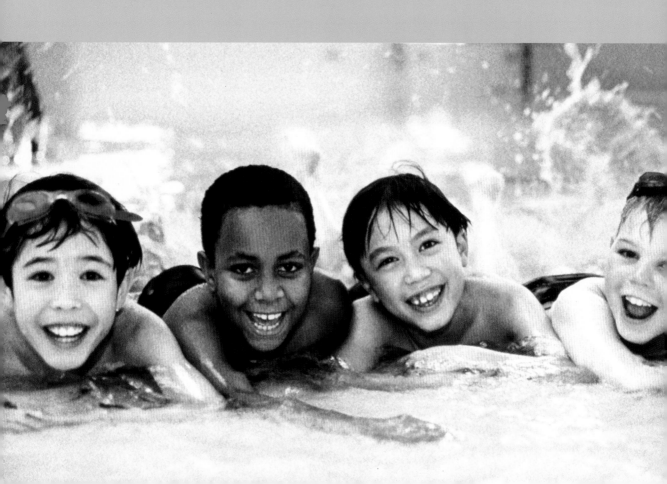

rude noises can be good for your face

As a result of watching children playing games with straws and drinks, I developed a range of exercises which I have used on my patients for many years to help them recover facial muscle strength after strokes and other neurological problems. Over the years I've seen that these simple exercises have cosmetic benefits too. They build excellent tone in your facial muscles which in turn support the structure of your skin. They also stimulate the blood flow to the cells of the skin and the skin's nerve supply. Making this small effort will repay you with a very large radiance dividend, so I strongly recommend these as a regular part of your ongoing radiance therapy. Repeat each exercise three times and try and repeat all 10 at least three times a week. Do them in front of you partner, children or grandchildren and everyone will have a good laugh as well, and as you know, laughter is the best medicine.

All you need are a large glass of water and a packet of thick plastic straws.

1 With the straw in the middle of your lips and the other end under the water, breathe in through your nose and very slowly out through the straw to produce a constant stream of bubbles.

2 Repeat as above, but with the straw in the left-hand corner of your mouth.

3 Repeat as above, but in the right hand-corner of your mouth.

4 Suck a mouthful of water through the straw as quickly as you can and swallow.

5 Suck a mouthful of water as slowly as you can and swallow.

6 Suck a mouthful of water and blow it back into the glass as quickly as you can.

7 Suck a mouthful of water and blow it back into the glass as slowly as you can.

8 Blow air through the straw into the water as hard as you can with your cheeks held in.

9 Blow air through the straw into the water as hard as you can with your cheeks puffed out.

10 Do this exercise in front of a mirror – raise your left eyebrow, raise your right eyebrow, purse your lips, blow a raspberry, suck in your cheeks, blow out your cheeks, blow another raspberry.

simple extras for added radiance

Throughout history, kitchen medicine has been the basis of healing. In the cauldrons of cave-dwellers, in the kitchens of priests, monks, medicine men, druids, alchemists and the village wise women, foods have been used both internally and externally for the treatment of virtually every ailment. Enhancing radiance is no exception and for many simple radiance-boosting applications you need look no further than your fridge, store cupboard, herb garden or greengrocer.

There are really considerable advantages when you make your own kitchen remedies to use on your skin, hands, nails and hair. Firstly, they are incredibly cheap. Secondly, you avoid the damaging chemical additives that are used in the vast majority of commercially available products, but thirdly, and most importantly, these kitchen remedies work better than most things that you buy over the counter from the pharmacy or the beauty shop – and you're not paying for all the excessive advertising or the environmentally damaging packaging.

Many of these DIY radiance products are simplicity itself– a jug of chamomile tea as a hair rinse, a bowl of warm olive oil to nourish the finger nails, garlic and vinegar to cure fungal infections, rosewater and glycerin for beautiful smooth hands, lemon juice to clean and whiten cuticles. You'll find how to use oats as one of the simplest of radiance-boosting skin nourishers and if you like chocolate, you'll discover a new use for it in this section of the book. There are even enzymes in pineapple which are good for your hands. And when it comes to hair the choice is endless. Apart from natural plant colourings, you can use artichoke, catmint, witch hazel or tea tree oil as a dandruff treatment, and you can even make your own shampoos for oily or dry hair.

Although hair and nails are extremely important when it comes to your total radiant look, it's the skin which most women worry about and this is where kitchen medicine really comes into its own. Cider vinegar, almonds, eggs, tomatoes and live yoghurt as well as fruits such as mangoes, peaches and avocados, and vegetables like cucumbers and cabbage, can all be made up into external applications for a wide variety of skin problems, ranging from dry skin, oily skin, spots and blemishes to acne, eczema and psoriasis. But this is just the tip of the iceberg. You can also use essential oils and fresh herbs to make steam infusions or to add to your bath, there are special honeys to treat infections, and the most effective remedy of all for boils is still the old-fashioned bread poultice which has been in regular use for at least 300 years.

I urge you to try these really simple radiance treats. They're fun to make, using them will give you the greatest of pleasure and you'll find that they really do work.

When it comes to supplements and extras to boost your radiance, I mostly recommend those that are based on natural products that have an inherent anti-inflammatory effect or that are rich in the plant hormones (phytoestrogens). These play a vital role in regulating hormonal balance, which is of particular importance for women who have irregular periods, suffer with Premenstrual Syndrome (PMS) or who are just beginning or have had the menopause. They are even more essential for women who have had a premature menopause, whether due to surgery, illness, anorexia or any other reason, as they may be the key to increased protection against osteoporosis, skin ageing and early heart disease.

kitchen remedies for skin

As we've already seen, eating lots of processed, packaged and convenience foods is certain to have an adverse effect on your skin, and alcohol and caffeine wreak havoc too. Obviously, the first thing to do is detox and improve your diet long-term, but meanwhile there are also some wonderful skin treatments you can produce in your very own kitchen.

live yoghurt and salt scrub

This is one of the simplest kitchen remedies for skin. Simply add 2 teaspoons of coarse sea salt to a carton of yoghurt, spread it evenly all over your face and leave for 10 minutes. Then, using cold water, gently rub the mixture all over the skin until it's rinsed off completely. The salt acts as a gentle exfoliator and antiseptic and the natural bacteria in the yoghurt provide a protective layer that will fight off any other bugs and help to prevent the formation of spots. It's worth doing this at least twice a week.

oats

These are a wonderful emollient for any inflamed skin. Put 4 tablespoons of uncooked oats in a muslin bag, hang the bag under the taps as you run the bath, then use the bag to clean your skin. The natural oils and vitamins in the oats will soothe inflamed areas and stimulate the growth of new skin. Use for 3 or 4 baths before replacing the oats.

avocados

These are nature's gift to the skin. They are not only wonderfully nutritious, but avocado oil makes a great skin food. After you've eaten your avocado, rub your skin with the inside of the peel and massage in the oily film that's left behind.

comfrey, calendula (from the marigold plant) and chamomile

These are three herbs which can easily be grown in your own garden and which have unique powers to soften, soothe, protect and heal the skin. Comfrey promotes the growth or regeneration of skin tissue; calendula clears up any infection – fungal, viral or bacterial – and counters inflammation; and chamomile soothes, heals and stimulates cell regeneration. Make up a strong infusion of all three, cool and strain it, then use it as a facial rinse or added to your bath.

oranges

These make a delicious face-mask. Purée the pulp of a whole orange, spread it over your face, leave for 20 minutes, then rinse off with tepid water. This leaves the skin feeling clean and stimulated. Your skin will also have absorbed some of the orange's vitamin C, betacarotene and a complex of bioflavonoids called vitamin P which strengthen the tiny capillaries, so protecting you from unsightly broken veins.

Face masks are also good made from honey, carrot grated into olive oil, and grape juice (or peeled and crushed fresh grapes)

lavender

This has been known for years to do wonders for the skin. Steep the tops of fresh lavender sprigs in white wine vinegar for a week (shake the bottle occasionally), then dilute 1 part of the vinegar to 4 parts of water and use as a skin tonic.

almond oil

This is used as a base for many natural skin products. You can make your own oil treatments by adding a couple of drops of your favourite essential oil to 1 tablespoon of almond oil. For oily skin, use chamomile, lavender or rose, while neroli or clary sage are good for older skins. Spread the oil mixture on your face and leave for 20 minutes, before washing off and applying a skin tonic.

fresh herbs

These are great for a facial sauna. Put a handful into a pan, pour boiling water over, cover the pan, leave to infuse for 10 minutes, then reheat. Remove from the heat, transfer to a heatproof bowl and lean over the steaming bowl with a towel over your head. Choose from lavender to heal and soothe the skin, rosemary to heal and stimulate the circulation, marigold to heal and cornflower to refresh. Mallow, marigold and sage are particularly good for problem skins, comfrey and borage flowers are great for dry skin and thyme will open your pores and get your blood really pumping.

kitchen remedies for hair

When your hair is looking less than radiant, it's often an early warning sign that you're not well. Your hairdresser will often notice a deterioration in the condition of your hair or scalp before any other symptoms appear. Once you've detoxed, you'll be well on the way to regaining a lovely head of hair, but some simple kitchen remedies can help too. And this isn't just for the ladies. Although men are much more likely to lose their hair, that's no excuse for not taking the best possible care of it while you can.

jojoba oil

This conditions and adds lustre to the hair. Heat a couple of tablespoons of jojoba oil, apply it to the roots, then comb it through the hair. Wrap a warm towel around your head and leave it for 30 minutes, then use a very mild shampoo to wash the oil out.

ginger root with sesame oil

Together these make a very stimulating conditioner. Squeeze the juice of the fresh root into a couple of tablespoons of oil, apply to the hair and wrap your head in a warm towel. Leave it on for as long as possible before shampooing.

rosemary

Traditionally used to stimulate local blood circulation. Add a handful to cold water, simmer for 15 minutes, then swab the roots of your hair with the mixture before shampooing.

nettles

Nettles are rich in the minerals needed for healthy growth. Try to wash your hair daily in a mild non-detergent nettle shampoo. Steam young nettletops to eat with a nob of butter and a little nutmeg, then use the steaming water to rub into your scalp.

onion

This is a wonderful source of sulphur, which is essential for healthy hair. As well as including onions in your diet, rubbing raw onion over the roots of your hair before you shampoo will stimulate your scalp.

for dandruff

Use a chamomile shampoo, and add a cup of cider vinegar to half a litre of hot water for the final rinse. In addition, massage your scalp thoroughly at bedtime with witch hazel extract or add a few drops of tea tree oil to your normal shampoo. You can also make a final rinse from a dozen or so globe artichoke leaves, simmered for 10 minutes, strained and cooled, or from catmint tea – a generous handful of chopped catmint leaves steeped in boiling water for 10 minutes, strained and left to cool.

for fair hair

To enhance blonde hair, make a final rinse from an infusion of mullein, strained and cooled, or from chamomile or from nettle teabag.

for dark hair

Condition with a solution of 1 cup of beetroot juice to 4 cups of hot water with a teaspoon of salt. Massage through the hair, then rinse out.

to cover grey

Avoid horrible commercial dyes yet cover your grey, by using sage. Add 4 large spoons of chopped leaves to a jug of boiling water, cover and leave for at least half an hour before straining. Use a brush or sponge to apply the liquid to the grey roots. Don't wash out.

for dry hair and flaky scalp

Warm a cup of olive oil in a bowl of hot water, massage it into the scalp and hair, wrap your head in a towel for 1 hour, then shampoo, and rinse with the chamomile and cider-vinegar mix (see above).

For dry hair on its own, add an egg yolk and a teaspoon of natural gelatin dissolved in a little boiling water to your favourite herbal shampoo.

for oily hair

To make the ideal shampoo for oily hair, mix together half a cup of rosewater, two whole eggs and a generous dash of dark rum.

kitchen remedies for nails and hands

You can be perfectly groomed from head to toe, but roughened skin on your hands and cracked, flaking, ridged or fungus-infected nails are impossible to hide. They can't help but detract from the radiant impression the rest of you is making. But never fear. Help is at hand as kitchen remedies once again come to your radiance rescue.

fungal nail infections

These are a common problem and very unsightly, but are easy to treat yourself. As I've already said, eat plenty of garlic for its powerful anti-fungal properties, but also bathe the affected nails in a mixture of a quarter of a litre of warm water, 15ml of cider vinegar and two crushed cloves of garlic. This will help athlete's foot as well.

brittle nails

Make sure you eat 10ml of extra-virgin olive oil each day and once a week soak your nails in a bowl of warm olive oil. After 10 minutes, wipe off the surplus. You can also strengthen your nails by soaking them in an infusion of dried horsetail.

reddened or chafed hands

Almonds and almond oil are kind to chafed hands. Make a soft paste of ground almonds and a little rosewater and spread it on your hands like a face mask. Leave on for about half an hour, then wipe off the surplus. Alternatively, mix together equal parts of rosewater and glycerin and rub into your hands at bedtime. You can wear soft cotton gloves during the night to boost the effect.

Essential oils also help rough hands. In a small bottle, mix 50ml of almond oil with 25 drops of chamomile, lavender or benzoin, and add a vitamin E capsule. Warm the bottle under a hot tap, then at bedtime, just massage the mixture in and sleep tight.

To prevent your hands getting rough in the first place, use a barrier cream for harsh or dirty jobs. In my opinion, the best is this one that you can make at home. Mix together 5g of kaolin (stocked by most chemists), 5g of cold-pressed almond oil and the yolk of 1 large organic egg. Rub the mixture well into the hands, particularly around the cuticles and under the nails and when you've finished your dirty tasks, simply scrub off with a soft bristle brush, leaving the hands clean and the skin soft and undamaged.

lemons

Always have fresh lemons in your kitchen. The flesh and juice rubbed into your hands not only help keep your hands clean but they whiten the skin, are strongly antiseptic and are an effective deodorant if you've been handling onions, garlic or fish.

oats

There's now a large range of oat-based commercial products for hand and skin care on the market, but save your money. Simply take a scoop of oats out of your porridge packet, put them in your cupped hand, add some water and rub your hands together until the oats form a paste. Massage this thoroughly in every nook and cranny of your hands, fingers, cuticles and nails, then rinse off. The fibre is an effective cleanser, but you also absorb vitamin E and other radiance-boosting nutrients through the skin.

chocolate

Sorry you don't get to eat it! But if you'd had a heavy session in the garden, been redecorating the house, or your job involves working with tools so you end up with calloused, hard hands, mix cocoa butter, beeswax and cold-pressed almond oil in equal proportions and heat them very slowly in a heatproof bowl over a saucepan of boiling water. When they've all dissolved together, remove from the heat and keep stirring until the mixture sets. Keep in a jam jar wrapped in foil and use as hand cream every night.

pineapple

Fresh pineapple contains the enzyme bromelaine which is a highly effective digestive enzyme that also softens the cuticles. Make a large glass of fresh pineapple juice, put 30ml into a jug with 3ml of cider vinegar and 5ml of extra-virgin olive oil. Whisk together and soak your nails for at least 15 minutes. Drink the rest of the juice!

supplements and natural remedies for lifelong radiance

I've already said it, but I'll say it again – no supplements are a substitute for healthy eating. But when it comes to radiance, there are a number of supplements and natural remedies that can provide a real boost. These are not 'magic bullets'. Think of them rather as an insurance that will give you the best possible chance of radiant good health when you're young, of feeling and looking great in your middle years, and of basking in that quiet glow of radiant energy, beautiful skin and healthy hair and nails which is especially important to our sense of self-esteem and well-being when we are older.

natural plant hormones

The natural plant hormones that can be extracted from soya beans, red clover and other plant material can be of major benefit in terms of maintaining and protecting your natural radiance. These are all available as supplements and as with virtually all medicines, finding the one that suits you best is a simple question of trial and error. They are particularly important in the treatment of acne, skin problems related to irregular periods, hormone imbalance, polycystic ovarian syndrome, adult acne, and at all stages of women's menopausal years – pre-, during and post-menopause.

essential fatty acids

These crop up time and time again as natural anti-inflammatories, for dealing with skin problems and for women's health problems in general, but there is now such an overwhelming body of scientific evidence that demonstrates their need, that they can't be ignored as a radiance protector and booster as well as for their more medicinal benefits.

Under this umbrella come the hugely beneficial cod-liver oil, fish oil, evening primrose oil, rapeseed oil and flax-seed oil. I'm afraid that the bad news for vegetarians and vegans is that there really is no substitute for the fish oils and though I know that most vegetarians and vegans would never eat oily fish, I really do urge them to take a supplement, especially if they're planning pregnancy or are pregnant or breastfeeding – if not for their own sake, then for that of their baby.

herbs and spices

Tried and tested through the years as radiance boosters, many herbs and spices are easy to grow or readily available in your supermarket, health food shop or greengrocer's.

parsley

This is a gentle diuretic which helps the body get rid of fluid. It's also rich in vitamins A and C, and is a reasonable source of iron. Make it into parsley tea (see page 16) and drink a glass every day. You'll find it's wonderful for the skin.

thyme

One of the most powerful anti-viral and anti-bacterial herbs, it protects against all forms of infection, particularly skin and stomach bugs. Add to tomato, cheese, egg or salad recipes.

cloves

A great aid to digestion and a help in the treatment of irritable bowel syndrome. Anything which improves digestive output means better skin and clearer eyes. Use it when cooking fruits and in stews and casseroles made from lamb, game or venison.

basil

A superb remedy for tension and anxiety headaches – a common cause of frowning and wrinkles – but it also has a gentle calming and soothing action which will help you relax and unwind. It's also useful in improving irregular periods.

sage

This is particularly important as we get older as sage helps to improve short-term memory and is also a strong protector against infections. For women approaching the menopause, sage helps even out hormone imbalances and reduces the risk of sudden ageing of the skin, breaking nails, hair loss and hot flushes. Use lots of it in cooking and drink a cup of sage tea daily – a teaspoon of chopped sage leaves to a cup of boiling water.

posture and colour for radiant looks

Stop and think for a moment about the last time you couldn't help but stare at someone in the street, getting out of a car or standing next to you at the supermarket checkout. You were no doubt wondering what made that person look so special. Regardless of age, sex or wealth, there are people whose radiance just shouts above the crowd. The fashion victims will tell you that these people have style, but that's not the reason they're so special. It's that indefinable combination of the way they move, their wonderful posture and deportment based on strong bones, and their innate sense of colour.

Few people make the link between radiance and posture but it is very real. We're all born with good posture. You only have to look at the way babies hold themselves when they first start to sit, crawl and walk. Their bodies achieve good posture naturally and with the minimum amount of effort. Unfortunately, though, learned behaviour soon takes over and thanks to badly designed furniture, acquired habits, sitting all day at a computer, lack of exercise and general laziness, our bodies suffer from chronic misalignment and we need a much greater muscular effort to hold ourselves up. This results in muscular tension and physical problems like head, neck, shoulder and low back pain. Often we have breathing and digestive difficulties too. Every movement we make drains our energy resources.

None of this contributes to our radiance. But for contrast, just think about those wonderful African and Asian women carrying bundles on their heads who seem to glide across the ground with such effortless grace. As you will see on the following pages, a combination of yoga, Alexander Technique and simple weight-bearing exercises can help you overcome your bad habits and relearn the art of graceful posture and movement.

The next step is to learn about the power of colour to unleash the new, radiant you. It's easy to scoff at the concept of colour therapy and to believe that it's a hangover from the hippy sixties or just the latest bit of twenty-first century psychobabble, but nothing could be further from the truth. Colour has been used as a mood-enhancing and therapeutic tool for at least two thousand years. Shamans, mystics, the physicians of ancient Greece, priests of almost every known religion, the great architects and artists of history and the psychiatrists of our modern age – all have discovered the immense power of colour.

In our own time, industrial psychologists advise companies on the best colours to use in offices, factories and workshops in order to enhance the work people do on these premises. And in the past, people who could afford it painted the rooms of their house in different colours according to the activities that went on there – reds for dining rooms to stimulate conversation and the intellect, greens for the library to aid concentration and calm when reading, the palest yellows for the most restful bedrooms, and terracotta and pinks for elegant, restrained sitting rooms.

Now we know that it's what you wear that matters too. As I'll show you, you can learn to dress for the occasion, so the colours you wear enhance the mood you need to feel and convey – whether it's for that special business meeting, for that interview for a new job, for a blind date or for a romantic dinner for two.

improve your posture

If you're trying to unlock your radiance, the key isn't simply to slap on more make-up in an attempt to cover up the flaws. Instead, you need to concentrate on improving your mobility, flexibility and bone strength. Fortunately, there are many tried and tested ways of doing this, ranging from yoga, Alexander technique and simple weight-bearing exercises that help keep the dreaded osteoporosis at bay.

yoga

Yoga is great for inner and outer radiance. It is a profoundly religious and spiritual system which has existed in India for thousands of years. In the west, it is mostly associated with a range of distinctive postures that promote mobility and flexibility and that also have therapeutic benefits for many parts of the body. Combining the postures with traditional yoga breathing helps establish patterns of profound relaxation and inner peace which can combat the lunatic pace of life that most of us live at in the twenty-first century.

Yoga is ideal for people of any age. You can learn the simple poses from books and videos but it's always best to learn from an experienced teacher who will ensure that you achieve the positions with the minimum effort and without risk of injury. For maximum benefit, once you're familiar with the postures, you need to practise on a daily basis.

alexander technique

Alexander was a struggling actor who discovered that his voice problems were caused by tension and bad posture. He developed his system to deal with these and over the years it has become hugely popular with dancers, musicians and performers of all kinds.

It offers a process of physical re-education that has far-reaching effects. For example, it can help with many conditions such as asthma, migraine, high blood pressure, backache and bowel problems. As far as your radiance is concerned, it will also help you move better so you look better, but even more importantly, it has a positive effect on your circulation and breathing. This will improve the oxygen-carrying ability of your blood which means more nutrients will be delivered to your skin.

Alexander is one technique that you cannot learn from books, videos or from the internet. Alexander practitioners think of themselves as teachers and their clients as pupils, and their job is to re-educate the postural bad habits that you've developed during your life. An Alexander teacher will gently realign your body to re-establish the perfect relationship between your head, neck and trunk. The technique also focuses on discovering how to use the minimum muscular effort required to achieve any single task. Through constant practice and learning to become aware of what you are doing, you will gradually come to feel uncomfortable with your bad old postural habits and will recognise what feels good and healthy.

weight-bearing exercise

One in three women and one in twelve men will develop osteoporosis and tragically it's happening in younger and younger people. Apart from eating a diet rich in calcium and vitamin D, the major protective factor against this life-destroying and ageing disease is weight-bearing exercise. Although most bone building goes on during the late teens, it's never too late to encourage your bones to strengthen themselves. You can get your exercise in any way that you enjoy, but you have to have your weight on your feet, so swimming and cycling don't count. A brisk 20-minute walk four times a week is all you need.

boost your radiance with colour

Do you automatically wear black, grey or beige clothes? Many of you will answer 'yes' and your excuse will be, 'because they're fashionable at the moment'. But did you know that colours like these that make you 'invisible' can also feed negative emotions such as sadness and depression? And once you're feeling down, you'll inevitably choose these colours, which means you're trapped in a downward spiral – none of which does your radiance any favours. But don't despair. There is a way out. Once you know a few tricks, you can use colour to your advantage in many situations – and give your radiance a boost at the same time.

Many colour therapy practitioners draw on elements of the ancient Indian art of Ayurvedic medicine and combine it with modern, scientific evidence. In Ayurvedic medicine, light and colour are regarded as two of the fundamental life forces which link the body's energy lines, or chakras. These, in turn, govern both our physical and our emotional state. Scientific evidence more or less supports this idea, suggesting that the whole spectrum of colours and wavelengths can have a profound effect on our mental and physical state.

As a general principle, scientific research tells us that red and yellow are the most strongly stimulating colours, while black and blue are the most calming. Many experiments have shown how changing a colour scheme can, for example, improve or reduce office productivity, performance on the factory floor children's learning ability, and people's physical and intellectual skills in a variety of situations.

A number of colour therapists also believe that every wavelength has its own vibrational frequency, which adds potency to the mix, but there's no scientific evidence to support this theory. Nevertheless, it's my experience that it doesn't matter whether you can see the colours you're wearing, the mere fact that you are wearing them is enough to change your mood – so perhaps it's the vibrations playing their part.

try it yourself

If you have to abide by a dress code at work, then add some splashes of colour. For example, if you're going to a meeting which you know will be stressful, women can try wearing a pale blue scarf or men a pale blue pocket handkerchief. This calming and soothing colour will help keep both your and your colleagues stress levels down.

For complex financial negotiations, when you know you'll need to concentrate hard, add some yellow – men can wear yellow braces, women yellow shoes or a yellow handbag. And if you know you're in for a very long and boring conference programme, then we're back to red. This stimulating colour will help keep you and those around you awake, and you'll still be looking good at the end of the day.

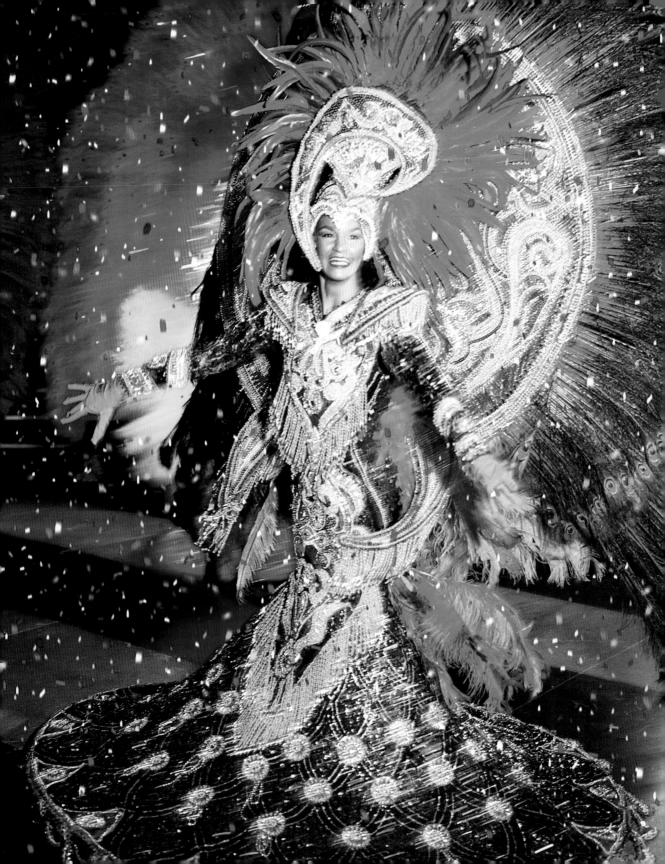

the strange case of margaret l.

I always note what colours my patients wear when they come to see me and I often surprise them in the middle of asking them the normal medical questions, by also asking them what their favourite colour is, what they wear to go to a dinner party or a dance, or what colour their favourite shirt is. In the case of Margaret L., it was the colour of her underwear that provided the key.

Unfortunately many people have to wear a uniform or some other approved form of dress for their job and it's one of these who is the unusual subject of this case history.

Like many people, Margaret had to follow a very rigid dress code at work. She was a 36-year old lawyer in a prestigious practice who first consulted me about a range of minor but uncomfortable gynaecological problems. After the second or third visit it soon became apparent that she was living life on the edge of anxiety, stress and depression, and I was seriously concerned she was about to have a breakdown. She was extremely clever and intelligent and could have been the most radiant person in any room, but she was in fact a drab, dull, boring mouse, with lifeless hair, grey skin and awful posture. Although she was well used to creating an impression in court, outside of her professional arena she paled into insignificance.

She was perfectly happy to talk about the physical and nutritional aspects of her health problems, but it took a while before she was even willing to admit that there were emotional problems. The truth was she hated the 'uniform' of black jacket, black skirt and black shoes that she had to wear at all times. She felt that it de-personalised her.

When I asked her what colour underwear she wore, she said it was usually grey – not much of a boost to anyone's morale or radiance. Since money was not a problem for her, I told her to go to the most expensive underwear shop she could find and buy three sets of red silk underwear. It took a while before she plucked up the courage to do it, but once she did it worked.

Over the next three months Margaret blossomed. Not only did her health improve, but the frog turned into a princess. She now radiates the inner beauty she always had but that was being held back by the straightjacket of her formal working clothes. And to the best of my knowledge, she's still wearing red knickers and hasn't looked back!

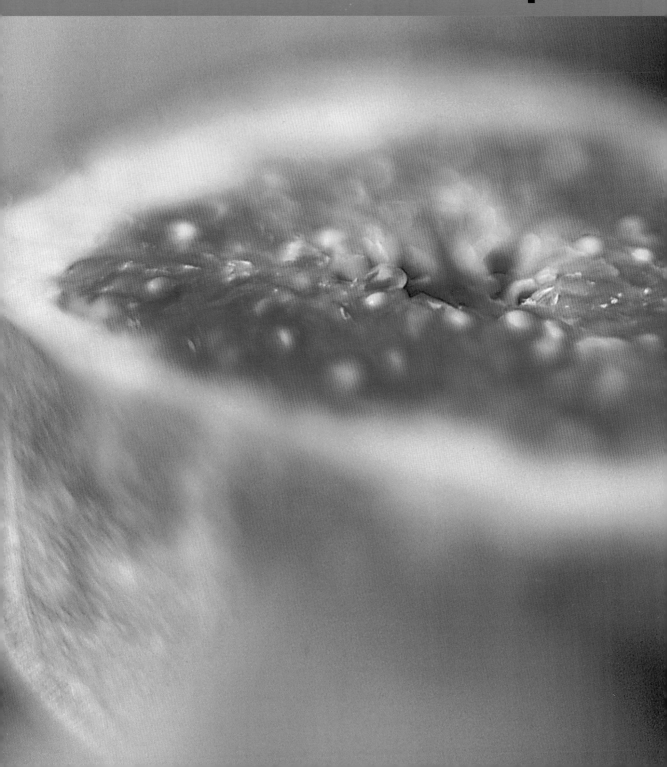

part 3

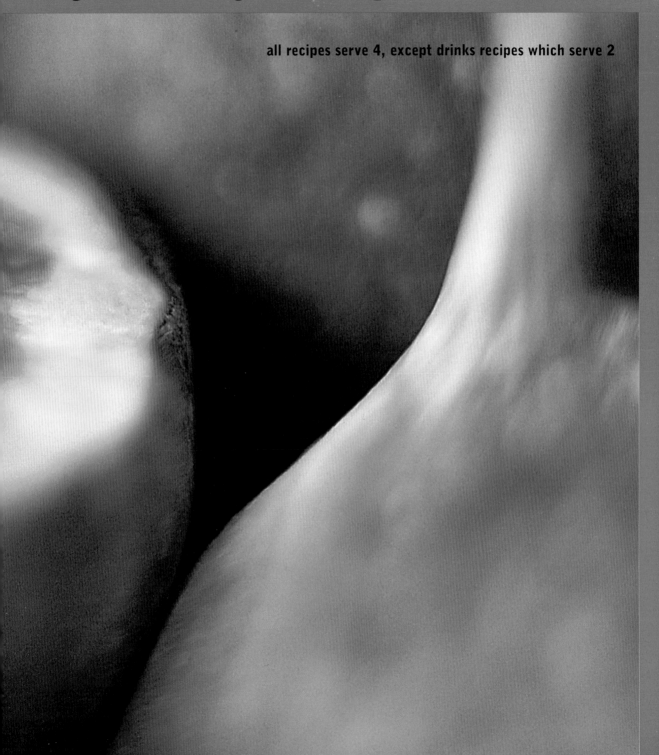

eat your way to super radiance

all recipes serve 4, except drinks recipes which serve 2

bread and breakfast

my easy bread

One of the most unhealthy modern myths is that bread is bad for you. In fact, this easy home-made bread is both an all-round health-giver and a super-radiance booster. It's especially rich in vitamins B and E – essential for healthy skin – as well as fibre to prevent constipation and encourage good digestion.

stoneground organic wholemeal bread flour	700g
easy-blend dried yeast	1 x 7g sachet
extra-virgin olive oil	2 tsp, plus extra for oiling
molasses, dark muscovado sugar or honey	1 tsp
salt	½ tsp
warm water	600ml
sunflower seeds (optional)	2 tbsp

Lightly oil a 1kg loaf tin and keep it warm. Mix the flour and yeast together in a large bowl. Dissolve the olive oil, molasses, sugar or honey and salt in the water. Make a well in the centre of the flour and pour in the warm water mixture and sunflower seeds, if using.

Mix all the ingredients together with a wooden spoon, then knead for about 4 minutes, until the dough forms a ball. Put it into the warm tin, cover with a damp tea towel and leave to rise in a warm place for about 40 minutes or until it has risen almost to the top of the tin. Meanwhile, preheat the oven to 200°C/400°F/Gas 6.

Transfer the tin to the preheated oven and bake for about 40 minutes, until it sounds hollow when you tap the bottom of the tin. When it's ready, remove from the oven and when it's cool enough to handle, transfer to a wire rack to cool completely.

cinnamon toast with figs

eggs	4
ground cinnamon	2 tsp
wholemeal bread	4 medium slices
butter	75g
dark brown sugar	2 tbsp
figs	4, fresh, halved lengthways, to serve

What a wonderful start to a leisurely day – and a great radiance boost too! The eggs in this delicious recipe contain iron, B vitamins and protein and there are cleansing essential oils in the cumin. Added to this, there's the ultimate pleasure of combining those delicious flavours with fresh figs, known since ancient times as one of nature's great skin foods.

Beat the eggs with half the cinnamon in a large bowl. Slice the bread into thick fingers. Melt the butter in a frying pan. Dip the bread in the egg mixture and fry in the butter on both sides until golden. Sprinkle with the brown sugar and extra cinnamon. Serve with the figs on the side.

radiance teabread

egg	1
chamomile tea	300ml made with 5 teabags and left to cool completely before the teabags are removed
dried dates	450g, chopped
soft brown sugar	200g
self-raising flour	250g

The calming effect of chamomile, and the iron and fibre in the dates makes this a delicious and extremely healthy snack for the odd moments of flagging energy.

Beat the egg. Put all the other ingredients in a large mixing bowl, add the beaten egg and mix well. Leave to stand for at least 6 hours. Preheat the oven to 180°C/350°F/Gas 4. Line a 1.2 litre loaf tin with greaseproof paper. Pour the mixture into the tin and bake in the preheated oven for 30 minutes. Turn out onto a wire rack and leave to cool.

colcannon

white cabbage	225g,
potatoes	450g, peeled and sliced
carrot	1, small, scrubbed and diced
turnip	1, small, thoroughly washed and thinly sliced
semi-skimmed milk	300ml
leek	1, small, thinly sliced
eggs	2, medium

An Irish chef on my radio programme once gave 'the definitive' recipe for colcannon. For the next three hours the phone rang as members of the London Irish community claimed they all had a better recipe. However, this is my favourite version, stolen from my wife's family in County Cavan. The sulphur in the cabbage, the vitamin A in the carrot, the minerals in the turnip and the anti-bacterial chemicals in the leeks are what I believe explain the sweet complexion that Irish girls are famous for.

Boil the cabbage until just tender, chop finely, then reserve until required. Meanwhile, boil the potatoes, carrots and turnips together until tender and mash coarsely.. Heat the milk in a saucepan, add the leek and simmer gently until tender. Drain the leek, reserving the milk and mash the cooked leek with the cooked cabbage into the potato mixture. Add enough of the leek milk to make a firm mash. Transfer to a casserole dish and grill under a preheated grill until golden on top. Meanwhile, poach the eggs and serve on top of the vegetable mixture.

drinks

Drinking enough fluid is always important, but it's an essential part of any detox plan as it helps flush out your body's toxins. But drinks can also provide the body with quickly and readily-absorbed nutrients, so what you drink is important. The recipes I give here are particularly abundant suppliers of super-radiance nutrients, so incorporate them in your daily living on a regular basis as well as using them where specified in the radiance detox plans.

As always, I recommend that you make your own juices from fresh, organic produce. It's not as difficult as you might think, but this really is the moment to invest in a good juicer or blender for your kitchen. As with everything, buy the best you can afford.

Most fruit and vegetables don't need peeling or coring, but you must remove any stones and thick skins, like the skin of pineapples and mangoes. Apart from that, just wash and cut into small enough pieces to fit into the machine. Once you get the hang of it, you'll be hooked and I'm sure you'll soon be experimenting with your own recipes before long.

tomato juice with garlic and spring onions

tomatoes	8, large,
spring onions	2 fat bulbs, trimmed
basil	4 large sprigs
oregano	6 large sprigs

Roughly chop the tomatoes and spring onions and put into a blender or liquidizer with the leaves from the basil and oregano. Whizz until smooth.

carrot, apple and celery juice

carrots	3, large
apples	2, quartered
celery	2 stalks

Peel the carrots if not organic, then simply cut everything into pieces and juice.

radiant juice

dessert apple	1, large quartered
orange	1, peeled, but with as much pith as possible
carrots	2, large, topped, tailed and peeled if not organic
fresh root ginger	2.5cm, peeled and sliced

This zingy juice full of vitamins A and C from the carrots and orange, soluble fibre for regular digestive function from the apple, and stimulating gingerole from the ginger will do more for your skin than a dozen pots of expensive cream. All these nutrients will improve the circulation, helping to carry health-giving nutrients directly to the skin.
Put the ingredients into a blender or liquidizer and whizz until smooth.

radiant lemonade

carrots	1, large, topped tailed and peeled if not organic
radishes	10, topped and tailed
apple	1, quartered
beetroot	1, topped and tailed
lemons	juice and finely grated zest of 2
naturally sparkling mineral water (optional)	up to 300ml

Vitamin A is essential for healthy, radiant skin and you'll get it in abundance from the carrots in this juice. The bonus comes from the radishes; their natural constituents stimulate the cleansing function of the liver, making this the perfect juice when you've been a bit over-indulgent or your digestive system seems slightly sluggish.
Juice the first 4 ingredients. Add the lemon juice and zest. If you want a longer, fizzy drink, add the mineral water.

soya blueberry and strawberry smoothie

blueberries	100g
strawberries	6, large
soya milk	425ml

Blueberries and strawberries on their own are super radiance boosters, but adding soya milk brings extra benefits. The natural plant hormones in soya help to regulate the hormonal seesaw of the menstrual cycle and also prevent some of the symptoms of the menopause. That makes this smoothie extremely female-friendly
Put the ingredients into a blender or liquidizer and whizz until smooth.

mango and soya milk smoothie

mango	1, large, ripe, cubed
soya milk	425ml

Put the ingredients into a blender or liquidizer and whizz until smooth.

yoghurt, papaya and kiwi smoothie

live natural yoghurt	500g
papaya	1, medium, peeled, pips removed, cubed
kiwi fruit	2, peeled and cubed

Put the ingredients into a blender or liquidizer and whizz until smooth.

kiwi and passion fruit smoothie

passion fruit	4
mascarpone cheese	250g
semi-skimmed milk	100ml
kiwi fruit	3, peeled and cut into chunks

Cut the passion fruit in half widthways and rub through a sieve to extract all the juice. Discard the pips. Put the rest of the ingredients into a blender or food processor and whizz until smooth. Alternatively, use a wand blender.

mango, kiwi and pineapple juice

mango	1, large, ripe and stoned
kiwi fruit	4
pineapple	1, medium, top and peel removed

The ultimate radiance drink, full of vitamins A, C and E, healing enzymes and a massive amount of natural plant chemicals.

Cut the ingredients into chunks, put in a blender or liquidizer and whizz until smooth.

carrot and beetroot juice

carrot	4, topped, tailed and peeled if not organic
beetroot	4, medium, preferably with leaves
basil	3 large sprigs

Put the ingredients into a blender or liquidizer and whizz until smooth.

lunches and dinners

prawn and tomato curry

onion	1, very finely chopped
tomatoes	1 x 400g can
garlic	1 clove, very finely chopped
coriander leaves	4 tbsp
frozen peas	75g
very veggie stock (see recipe page 96)	200ml
ground coriander	1 tsp
ground cumin	1 tsp
sun-dried tomato paste	2 tbsp
curry powder	1 tsp
fresh red chilli	1, deseeded and very finely chopped
cooked peeled prawns	400g
crème fraîche	1 x 200g tub
cooked rice	to serve

This is a variation on traditional kedgeree. It overflows with a combination of protective nutrients which will boost and enhance your radiance.

Put the onion, tomatoes, garlic, half the fresh coriander, the peas and the stock in a large saucepan and simmer for 5 minutes. Mix together the ground coriander, cumin, tomato paste, curry powder and chilli. Add to the stock and simmer for a further 5 minutes. Add the prawns and simmer for 3 minutes. Sprinkle with the remaining fresh coriander, stir in the crème fraîche and serve on a bed of rice.

potted shrimps

unsalted butter	150g
allspice	2 tsp
lemon	juice of ½
shrimps	600g, peeled weight, thoroughly thawed if bought frozen
bay leaves	3

Melt the butter in a medium saucepan. Add the allspice and lemon juice and leave to rest, off the heat, for 10 minutes. Put the shrimps into a 700ml shallow pot. Strain the butter over them, pushing them down so that all the shrimps are covered. Push in the bay leaves, making sure they're covered by the butter, too. Cover and leave to cool in the fridge until the butter solidifies – at least 1 hour.

ratatouille

extra-virgin olive oil	6 tbsp
onions	2, large, finely chopped
garlic	4 cloves, finely chopped
green peppers	2, large, deseeded and finely chopped
aubergine	1, large, finely cubed
chopped tomatoes	1 x 400g can

Heat the olive oil and sauté the onions and garlic gently for 5 minutes in a large saucepan. Add the peppers and aubergine and continue to sauté for a further 5 minutes. Add the tomatoes, cover the pan and simmer gently for 30 minutes.

stir-fried turkey breast with vegetables and noodles

egg noodles	400g
rapeseed oil	2 tbsp
fresh root ginger	2.5cm, grated
garlic	10 cloves, peeled
chilli	1, red, deseeded and finely chopped
turkey breast	450g, finely cubed
onion	1, small, finely chopped
mixed vegetables	450g finely chopped baby carrots, broccoli, mangetout, sweetcorn, cauliflower, cabbage, or a packet of stir-fry vegetables
sesame oil	2 tbsp
soy sauce	1 tbsp

Turkey is a good source of protein and essential B vitamins, but is virtually fat-free. Mixed here with the skin-nourishing root vegetables and circulation-stimulating ginger and chilli, this is an all-year-round radiance-enhancing recipe.

Cook the noodles according to the packet instructions. Meanwhile, heat the oil in a preheated wok or large saucepan and stir-fry the ginger, garlic, chilli and turkey for 2 minutes. Add the onion and vegetables and stir in the sesame oil. Stir-fry for a further 4 minutes, adding the soy sauce gradually, until the vegetables are just beginning to crisp. Remove from the heat. Drain the cooked noodles, mix into the stir-fry and serve immediately.

eggs florentine

baby spinach	900g
unsalted butter	50g
plain flour	3 tbsp
semi-skimmed milk	124ml
tarragon	4 large sprigs, leaves removed and chopped
eggs	4, large

Preheat the oven to 170°C/325°F/ Gas 3. Wash the spinach, even if the packet says it's ready-washed. Put into a saucepan with just the water clinging to it. Add half the butter, cover the pan and cook over a low heat until wilted, about 5 minutes. Divide between 4 medium ramekin dishes.

Heat the remaining butter in a small saucepan, add the flour and milk and cook gently until you have a roux. Reduce the heat to minimum, add the tarragon and simmer for 3 minutes. Put half the mixture into the ramekins. Crack an egg into each. Top with the rest of the tarragon sauce and bake in the preheated oven for 20 minutes.

salmon fishcakes with tomato salsa

crushed tomatoes	2 x 400g cans
garlic	4 cloves, finely chopped
red chillies	2, deseeded and finely chopped
capers	2 tbsp, rinsed
rapeseed oil	100 ml
onion	1, finely chopped
salmon	1 x 200g can, drained
wholemeal breadcrumbs	6 tbsp
dill	2 tbsp freshly chopped leaves
parsley	2 tbsp freshly chopped leaves
eggs	2, beaten

Make the tomato salsa by putting the first 4 ingredients in a blender and whizzing until smooth. Set aside until required.

Heat 2 tbsp of the oil in a saucepan and sauté the onion gently until golden, about 5 minutes. Meanwhile, put the fish in a bowl and mash with a fork. Mix with the breadcrumbs, dill and parsley and mix in the egg. Using your hands, make into tangerine-sized mounds and flatten to about 1cm thick. Heat the remaining oil in a frying pan and fry the fish for 3 minutes on each side until golden. Serve with the salsa.

potato cakes with broccoli

potatoes	800g, peeled and grated
eggs	2
broccoli	150g small florets
onion	1, medium, finely chopped
parsley	3 tbsp finely chopped leaves
garlic	2 cloves, finely chopped
rapeseed oil	5 tbsp
plain flour	2 tbsp

In this posh form of bubble and squeak, it's the broccoli that adds the super-radiant nutrients. This is a great way to encourage spotty adolescents to eat their greens.

Mix together the potatoes, eggs, broccoli, onion, parsley and garlic. Heat the oil in a large frying pan and add the potato mixture, flatten with a fork and sprinkle the flour on top. Cook over a medium heat until the bottom is golden, about 10 minutes. Preheat the grill to hot and transfer the frying pan to it. Cook until the top is golden. Slide the potato cakes onto kitchen paper to soak up any excess oil, then onto a plate to serve.

grilled sole with cheese

sole fillets	4
salt and pepper	to season
unsalted butter	50g
Dijon mustard	4 tsp
Cheddar cheese	4 tbsp, grated

Season the fillets with salt and pepper. Preheat the grill to its highest setting and line a grill pan with kitchen foil. Brush the foil with the butter, then put the fillets on top. Put under the grill and turn immediately. Brush with the mustard, sprinkle on the cheese and return to the grill until the fish is cooked, about 3 minutes.

quick chickpea casserole

olive oil	4 tbsp
onion	1, finely chopped
garlic	3 cloves, finely chopped
tomatoes	1 x 400g can
chickpeas	1 x 400g can
frozen mixed vegetables	450g
bouquet garni	1 sachet
stock	900ml
parsley	2 tbsp freshly chopped leaves

Cheap, filling, easy to use but much ignored, chickpeas are an excellent radiance food. Apart from their cleansing fibre and B vitamins, they also contain minerals essential for maintaining the structure and elasticity of the skin.

Heat the olive oil in a large saucepan and sauté the onion and garlic gently until just soft. Pour in the tomatoes with their juice and bring to a simmer. Meanwhile, drain and rinse the chickpeas. Add the chickpeas, mixed vegetables, bouquet garni sachet and stock to the onion and garlic mixture and simmer for 15 minutes. Sprinkle with the chopped parsley and serve.

lentil and barley pilaff

pot-barley	125g
very veggie stock	600ml
(see recipe page 96)	
brown lentils	225g
olive oil	4 tbsp
carrot	1, finely chopped
celery	1 stick, finely chopped
onions	2, sliced
parsley	1 tbsp freshly chopped
	leaves
live natural yoghurt	175g

Wash the barley, soak in cold water to cover for 1 hour and drain. Put the stock into a large saucepan, add the barley and simmer, covered, for 45 minutes or until tender. Meanwhile, cook the lentils according to the packet instructions (this normally takes 30–40 minutes). Heat 1 tbsp of the oil in a frying pan and sauté the carrot, celery and half the onions gently for 4 minutes. Mix with the barley and lentils and keep warm in a 180°C/350°F/Gas 4 oven. Heat the rest of the oil in a frying pan and fry the remaining onion. Serve the pilaff garnished with the onion rings and parsley and with the yoghurt on the side.

chicken liver kebabs

wooden skewers	4
chicken livers	250g
unsalted butter	110g
shallots	4, very finely
	chopped
sage leaves	12
brown-cap mushrooms	8, stems removed
cherry tomatoes	12, halved
red peppers	1, deseeded and
	cubed

Another recipe for outer and inner radiance. The chicken livers are full of iron and B vitamins for healthy blood, there's lycopene in the tomatoes, betacarotene and vitamin C in the peppers, and the bonus of mind-boosting essential oils in the sage.

Soak the skewers in water for 30 minutes before using to prevent burrning. Preheat the grill and line a grill rack with foil. Wash and dry the chicken livers, cutting off any membranes. Heat half the butter in a saucepan and sauté the chicken livers and shallots for 2 minutes, stirring continuously. Remove with a slotted spoon and keep warm. Add the sage leaves to the pan and sauté until slightly crisp. Remove and keep warm. Thread the chicken livers onto the kebab sticks, alternating them with the remaining ingredients. Brush each kebab with the remaining butter and cook under the preheated grill for 5 minutes, turning once. Alternatively, cook on a barbecue.

stuffed green peppers

green lentils, preferably Puy	300g, washed
green peppers	4, large
extra-virgin olive oil	4 tbsp
onion	2, finely chopped
garlic	3 cloves, finely chopped
Worcestershire sauce	2 tbsp
Cheddar cheese	200g, grated

Cook the lentils according to the packet instructions (this normally takes 30–40 minutes). Preheat the oven to 180°C/350°F/Gas 4. Meanwhile, halve the peppers widthways, deseed and put into a large baking tin, add 2.5cm of water and bake in the preheated oven for 40 minutes. While they are cooking, heat the oil in a saucepan and sauté the onion and garlic until soft. Drain the lentils, reserving 4 tbsp of their cooking liquid, and mix this liquid together with the lentils and Worcestershire sauce into the onion and garlic. Pile the mixture into the peppers. Sprinkle with the cheese and return to the oven for 15 minutes.

courgette pasta

thin pasta, such as spaghettini	400g
courgettes	4 medium, grated
fresh root ginger	3cm, grated
light soy sauce	2 tbsp
extra-virgin olive oil	4 tsp
Parmesan cheese	4 tsp, freshly grated
spring onion	4, finely chopped
beansprouts	125g

Cook the pasta in a saucepan of boiling water according to the packet instructions. Transfer to a large serving bowl and mix in all the other ingredients. Serve immediately.

tomato risotto

extra-virgin olive oil	4 tbsp
onion	1, finely chopped
garlic	2 cloves, finely chopped
brown rice	225g
sun-dried tomatoes	175g, drained if in oil
very veggie stock (see recipe page 96)	800ml
tomatoes	4
basil	12 fresh leaves, roughly torn
Parmesan cheese	3 tbsp, freshly grated

Heat the oil in a saucepan and sauté the onion and garlic gently until soft. Add the rice, chopped sun-dried tomatoes and stock. Peel the tomatoes by putting them in a bowl and covering them with freshly boiled water. Leave to stand for a few minutes until until the skins split, then peel, chop them and add to the pan. Simmer for 40 minutes. Stir in the basil and cheese just before serving.

pasta with tuna fish and black olives

Quicker than queuing at a take-away, the olives and their oil in this 15-minute recipe provide plenty of skin-nourishing vitamin E and mono-unsaturated fat, while the fish contains anti-inflammatory essential acids. In addition, there's an energy boost from the pasta.

Put the tomatoes, with their juices, into a large saucepan. Add the crumbled stock cube, wine, onion, olive oil and chilli. Simmer for 10 minutes and add the herbs. Mix in the tuna and olives. Heat through gently while you cook the pasta in a large saucepan according to the packet instructions. Stir the sauce into the pasta and serve.

tomatoes	1 x 400g can
vegetable stock cube	1
white wine	2 tbsp
onion	1, very finely chopped
olive oil	2 tbsp
chilli	1, red or green, deseeded and finely chopped
parsley, basil and coriander, mixed	1 tbsp, freshly chopped
tuna	1 x 200g can, in oil, drained and flaked
olives	10, black, stoned
pasta	250g

tofu, vegetable and cashew nut stir-fry

This is the ultimate radiant meal, with natural plant hormones from the tofu, antibacterial sulphur from the cabbage, masses of vitamin A from the carrots and more than your day's requirement of vitamin C.

Heat the oil in a preheated wok, add the tofu and fry gently until golden brown. Remove from the wok with a slotted spoon and reserve. Add the onion, green pepper, ginger and celery and sauté gently until soft. Add the carrots and cabbage and sauté for 4 minutes. Add the mushrooms and cashew nuts and cook for a further 1 minute. Pour in the stock, cover and simmer until the vegetables are soft. Just before serving, add the fried tofu and the soy sauce.

olive oil	3 tbsp
tofu	250g, drained and cubed
onion	1, finely chopped
green pepper	1, deseeded and cubed
fresh root ginger	1cm, grated
celery	1 stalk, finely sliced
carrots	2, medium, finely sliced
cabbage	½ shredded
mushrooms	100g, wiped and sliced
cashew nuts	125g
very veggie stock (see recipe page 96)	200m
soy sauce	1 tsp

bean casserole

olive oil	1 tsp
onion	1, finely chopped
garlic	2 cloves, finely chopped
chilli powder	1 tbsp
mustard powder	1 large pinch
white wine vinegar	2 tbsp
tomato purée	1 tbsp
Worcestershire sauce	1 tsp
tomatoes	1 x 200g can, crushed
very veggie stock (see recipe page 96)	500ml
root vegetables	900g mixed carrots, swedes, parsnips, turnips etc, all diced
mushrooms	125g, sliced
chickpeas	1 x 200g can
borlotti beans	1 x 200g can

The beans in this delicious casserole are a source of natural plant hormones, which give a brilliant radiance boost. With the betacarotene and minerals from the root vegetables and masses of cancer-protective and skin-nourishing lycopene from the tomatoes, this is a wonderful meal for chilly autumn or winter evenings. And the leftovers are even nicer heated up the following day.

Heat the oil in a large saucepan and sauté the onion and garlic until soft. Add the chilli, mustard and vinegar and simmer for 1 minute. Mix in the tomato purée, Worcestershire sauce, tomatoes and stock. Add the root vegetables and simmer for 20 minutes until tender. Add the mushrooms, drained and rinsed chickpeas and beans, and cook for a further 5 minutes.

scrambled eggs with smoked mackerel

smoked mackerel fillets	225g, flaked
single cream	3 tbsp
lemon	juice of ½
spring onions	4, large, finely chopped
butter	50g
eggs	6
parsley	2 tbsp finely chopped leaves
wholemeal toast	to serve

The perfect radiance recipe. The essential fatty acids in the fish are nature's most effective anti-inflammatories, while the iron and lecithin in the eggs help prevent the pallor of anaemia and stimulate skin cell growth.

Mix the mackerel fillets with the cream, lemon juice and spring onions in a large bowl. Set aside. Heat the butter in a non-stick frying pan. Add the eggs and gently break up the yolks. Continue cooking, pushing the egg mixture in from the outside of the pan – you want the yolks and whites to stay slightly separate. When the eggs are beginning to set, add the mackerel mixture and stir until you have the consistency you prefer. Scatter with the parsley leaves and serve immediately with wholemeal toast.

griddled tuna with roasted vegetables and fusilli

extra-virgin olive oil	100ml
rosemary	1 large sprig
garlic	2 cloves, finely chopped
tuna steaks	4
rapeseed oil	100ml
peppers	1 red, 1 green, deseeded and cut into thick strips
onions	2, quartered
courgettes	4, small, halved lengthways
fennel	1 bulb, quartered lengthways
baby leeks	2, halved lengthways
fusilli	400g

Fresh tuna is an excellent source of radiant-boosting essential fatty acids, and the fennel, with its hint of liquorice flavour, helps to stimulate the cleansing functions of the liver. This is a versatile dish that you can also cook under a hot grill or on a summer barbecue.

Put the olive oil, rosemary and garlic into a large, shallow dish. Add the tuna and coat in the mixture. Cover and leave in the fridge. Meanwhile, preheat the oven to 220°C/425°F/Gas 7. Put the rapeseed oil into a baking dish, add the vegetables and stir to coat well. Roast in the preheated oven for 30 minutes, stirring occasionally. When the vegetables are nearly ready, cook the fusilli in a large saucepan of boiling water according to the packet instructions. Preheat a griddle pan. Remove the tuna from the marinade, leaving some of the oil still clinging, and cook in the griddle pan over a high heat for 2 minutes on each side. Serve in a mound, with the fusilli on the bottom, then the vegetables and the tuna on top.

sage burgers

mixed nuts	225g
wholemeal breadcrumbs	110g
sunflower oil	about 125ml
onion	1, medium, very finely chopped
very veggie stock (see recipe page 96)	300ml
yeast extract	2 tsp
sage	6 leaves, finely chopped
wholemeal flour	4 tbsp, for dusting

These are a highly nutritious alternative to meat-based burgers, and with the bonus that they contain no saturated fat. Added to that, they are rich in skin-friendly minerals, especially zinc and selenium, and have lots of fibre, which encourages good digestion. The nuts also provide radiance-enhancing vitamin E.

Grind the nuts and breadcrumbs in a food processor or blender. Heat 2 tbspns of the oil in a saucepan and sauté the onion gently until soft. Heat the stock and yeast extract together in a separate saucepan until blended. Mix the ground nuts, breadcrumbs and onion together, adding enough of the stock and yeast extract mixture to make a good consistency. Shape into 4 burgers and dust with the flour. Heat the rest of the oil in a large frying pan and shallow-fry the burgers for 4 minutes on each side.

beef and ginger stir-fry

cornflour	1 tbsp
Chinese five-spice powder	½ tsp
soy sauce	3 tbsp
lean grilling steak – fillet is best	400g cut into thin strips
sesame oil	3 tbsp
fresh root ginger	2cm, grated
garlic	2 cloves, very finely chopped
red pepper	1, small, deseeded and finely cubed
broccoli	1 medium head, florets removed and stalks finely sliced
spring onions	4, sliced diagonally
sherry	½ an average glass
cooked rice or noodles	to serve

Mix the cornflour, Chinese five-spice powder and soy sauce together in a large bowl. Add the steak and stir to coat thoroughly. Cover and leave to marinate in the fridge for about 20 minutes. Heat the oil in a preheated wok or large frying pan and add the steak, ginger and garlic. Stir-fry for 4 minutes. Add the pepper, broccoli florets and stalks and spring onions, and continue cooking for a further 2 minutes. Pour in the sherry, cover the pan and cook for 1 minute. Serve with rice or noodles.

one-pot pasta with vegetables and pesto

spaghetti	400g
french beans	75g, finely chopped
courgettes	2, finely diced
new potatoes	3, very finely diced
pesto sauce	4 tbsp
Parmesan cheese	3 tbsp, freshly grated

Another quick, easy and inexpensive meal with minimum effort and maximum benefit. As well as the skin-friendly nutrient in the vegetables, there's added value from the mood-enhancing essential oils in basil.

Bring a large saucepan of water to the boil and add the spaghetti and vegetables. They will all be just tender at the same time, about 6 minutes. Drain, reserving 2 tsp of the water and mix this in a bowl with the pesto. Mix the pesto with the drained pasta and vegetables. Add the Parmesan and serve immediately.

baked halibut with mushrooms

unsalted butter	about 50g
halibut steaks	4
shallots or small onions	3, very finely chopped
oyster mushrooms	150g, wiped and sliced
dry white wine	100ml
lemon	juice of ½
parsley	2 tbsp freshly chopped leaves

Preheat the oven to 190°C/375°F/Gas 5. Rub half the butter over the base of a large, shallow ovenproof dish and put the halibut in it. Melt the rest of the butter and sauté the shallots and mushrooms gently until soft. Cover the fish with the shallots and mushrooms, pour over the wine and bake in the preheated oven for 20–25 minutes. Sprinkle over the lemon juice and parsley and serve.

non-meatballs in tomato sauce

vegeburger mix	450g
garlic	3 cloves, finely chopped
mint	2 tbsp freshly chopped leaves
parsley	2 tbsp freshly chopped leaves
tomatoes	1 x 400g can
vegetable stock cube	1
white wine	4 tbsp
onion	1, large, finely chopped
extra-virgin olive oil	1 tbsp
green chilli	1, deseeded and finely chopped
rapeseed oil	100ml

There's a double radiance bonus in this dish, which comes from the radiant-friendly nutrients in the vegeburger mix and also from the lycopene in the tomatoes. Lycopene is one of the most powerful natural protective anti-oxidants. It also stimulates new skin cell growth, slows the skin's ageing process and is a mighty wrinkle-zapper.

Prepare the vegeburger mix according to the packet instructions, adding the garlic, mint and parsley. Put the tomatoes and their juice into a large frying pan with the crumbled stock cube, wine, onion, olive oil and chilli. Bring to the boil and simmer for 10 minutes. While the sauce is cooking, form the vegeburger mixture into walnut-sized balls and fry gently in the rapeseed oil for 3 minutes on each side. Add them to the tomato sauce and serve immediately.

chicken with thyme and lemon

wholemeal flour	3 tbsp
dried thyme	2 tsp
chicken thighs	8
milk	100ml
rapeseed oil	4 tbsp
lemon	juice of 1

Preheat the oven to 190°C/375°F/Gas 5. Mix the flour and thyme together in a large bowl. Dip the chicken in the milk and roll in the flour mixture. Heat the oil in large frying pan and fry the chicken until browned on all sides. Transfer the chicken to a wire rack placed over a roasting tin and pour over the lemon juice. Bake in the preheated oven for 15 minutes.

risotto con salsa cruda

This rice and raw vegetable dish provides nutrients at their best. None of the essential ingredients are lost in cooking, which means you get optimum radiance benefits with minimum effort.

cucumber	1, peeled, deseeded and finely cubed
tomatoes	4, coarsely chopped
spring onions	4, finely sliced
garlic	2 cloves, finely chopped
carrots	4, very finely cubed
radishes	4, halved
courgettes	3 small, finely cubed
fresh peas	50g
extra-virgin oilve oil	4 tbsp
long-grain brown rice	250g
chives	1tbsp, snipped
parsley	1 tbsp freshly chopped leaves

Put the vegetables in a bowl, mix in the oil and leave to marinate for half an hour. Meanwhile, cook the rice according to the packet instructions. Remove from the heat and leave uncovered for 10 minutes to dry and separate. Drain if necessary. While the rice is still warm, mix it into the mixed vegetables and sprinkle on the herbs.

grilled paprika chicken

paprika	1 tsp
freshly ground black pepper	2 good twists
lemon	juice and grated rind of 1
rapeseed oil	4 tbsp
garlic	2 cloves, very finely chopped
chicken breasts	4, skinless and boneless, flattened

Mix the paprika, pepper, lemon, oil and garlic together in a bowl. Put the chicken breasts in a large, shallow dish and pour over the marinade. Cover and leave in the fridge for at least 1 hour. Preheat the grill and line a grill pan with foil. Remove the chicken from the marinade and place on the grill rack. Cook under the preheated grill for 6–7 minutes on each side, depending on thickness, basting occasionally with the marinade.

pitta bread pizza

wholemeal pittas	4
tomatoes	4, sliced
dried oregano	1 tsp
Cheddar cheese	4 tbsp grated
extra-virgin olive oil	4 tsp

Preheat the grill to high and toast the pittas on one side for 1 minute. Turn them over, arrange the tomatoes on top, sprinkle with the oregano, then the cheese. Drizzle the oil on top and return to the grill until the cheese is bubbling, about 2 minutes.

soups and salads

Chemical pollution is the major enemy of radiance. You can't do much about environmental pollutants, but there's a great deal you can do to reduce your consumption of radiance-destroying toxins. One of the most satisfying steps is to steer clear of extremely expensive ready-made salad dressings and to throw away stock cubes, gravy granules and all the other instant solutions – and instead, make your own. Take this simple step and you'll get an abundance of all the radiance nutrients with their healing and protective properties.

very veggie stock

onions	2; 1 peeled and quartered, 1 left whole
celery	3 large stalks, with their leaves
leeks	1
parsnip	1
sage	1 large sprig
thyme	2 sprigs
bay leaves	6
parsley	2 generous handfuls
peppercorns	12, black, whole
water	2 litres

This basic recipe may seem as if it takes a long time and will leave you with far more stock than you need. But it's simple to make and healthier than any commercial stock or cube. If you don't need all of it, you can boil it down until it has reduced to half its volume, put it into the freezer – I often freeze it in ice-cube trays – then add it to an equal amount of boiling water and use as required. Put all the ingredients into a large saucepan, cutting them to fit if necessary. Bring slowly to the boil and simmer for 40 minutes. Strain and use as required.

Put all the ingredients into a large saucepan, cutting them to fit the space if necessary. Bring slowly to the boil and simmer for 40 mins. Strain and use as required.

my salad dressing

extra-virgin olive oil	300ml
white wine vinegar	100ml
Dijon mustard	1 tbsp
spring onions	2, very finely chopped
garlic	1 clove, very finely chopped
parsley	1 tsp chopped leaves

Mix all the ingredients together in a bowl. Transfer to a screw-topped jar and shake well. Serve. This will keep for up to 2 weeks, unrefrigerated.

basic chicken stock

chicken	1 carcass – the remains of the Sunday roast will do, but it's better to ask a butcher to keep a carcass which has been stripped of its other useful meat.
water	2 litres
spring onions	6, with the stems on
leeks	1, large, trimmed and coarsely chopped
celery	2 large stalks, chopped
rosemary	1 large sprig
parsley	2 generous handfuls
sage	1 large sprig
thyme	2 large sprigs
bay leaves	3
peppercorns	10, white

Put the chicken carcass into a large heavy-based saucepan and cover with the water. Bring to the boil and cook, uncovered, for 30 minutes. Add the rest of the ingredients, partially cover the pan and simmer for 40 minutes, adding more water if necessary. Strain and use as required.

sweetcorn and haddock chowder

smoked haddock	350g
semi-skimmed milk	700ml
bay leaves	2
unsalted butter	50g
onion	1, large, very finely chopped
garlic	1 clove, very finely chopped
potatoes	225g, peeled and finely cubed
sweetcorn	200g, frozen or canned
single cream	300ml

At first sight you may wonder what this soup has to offer for radiance, but the fish is a rich source of iodine, lack of which can lead to dry, lifeless hair, coarseness of the skin and chronic exhaustion. Iodine is also essential for the normal function of the thyroid gland, which controls the body's metabolism, so that's an important bonus.

Poach the haddock in the milk, with the bay leaves, for about 5 minutes. Remove the bay leaves and discard. Remove the fish with a slotted spoon and flake the flesh with a fork. Reserve the poaching liquid. Heat the butter in a saucepan and sauté the onion and garlic gently until soft. Add the potatoes and the reserved poaching liquid and simmer until tender. Add the sweetcorn, then stir in the fish and cream and heat through for 5 minutes or until the sweetcorn is tender. Serve immediately.

chilled avocado soup

avocados	5, ripe
very veggie stock (see recipe page 96)	1 litre
lemon	juice of 1
garlic	2 large cloves, finely chopped
red chillies	2, deseeded and chopped
cayenne pepper	½ tbsp
spring onions	5, roughly chopped
tomatoes	1 x 200g can
live natural yoghurt	150g
pumpkin seed	25g

The ultimate for inner and outer radiance, offering the legendary skin benefits of avocados, which are rich in vitamin E and antioxidants, the circulation-boosting properties of chilli and cayenne pepper, the protective bacteria in the yoghurt and lots of zinc from the pumpkin seeds.

Put the avocado flesh into a food processor or large blender with the next 7 ingredients and whizz until smooth. Add the yoghurt and whizz again for a few seconds. Spoon into a bowl and leave to cool in the fridge. Dry-fry the pumpkin seeds in a small frying pan. Remove the pan from the heat and leave to cool. Sprinkle the pumpkin seeds on the soup just before serving.

watercress soup

Watercress is one of the truly great radiant foods. It's hugely antioxidant, especially protective against lung cancer and rich in iron, which makes it a key to inner beauty.

Heat the oil in a large saucepan and sauté the onion gently until soft. Add the garlic and continue to cook for 2 minutes. Add the watercress and continue to cook gently until it wilts. Add the stock and simmer for about 10 minutes. Transfer to a blender or food processor and whizz until smooth. Serve hot or cold with a swirl of yoghurt in each bowl.

olive oil	1 tbsp
onion	1, medium, finely chopped
garlic	2 cloves, finely chopped
watercress	3 bunches, with stalks
very veggie stock (see recipe page 96)	1 litre
live natural yoghurt	200g

spinach soup with yoghurt

Heat the oil in a saucepan and sauté the onion and garlic gently until soft. Add the spinach, mint and stock and simmer for 10 minutes. Transfer the soup to a blender or food processor and whizz until smooth. Serve with a swirl of yoghurt and the nutmeg on top.

rapeseed oil	2 tbsp
onion	1, finely chopped
garlic	2 cloves, finely chopped
fresh or frozen spinach	900g
mint	3 tender sprigs
very veggie stock (see recipe page 96)	1 litre
live natural yoghurt	200g
nutmeg	4 pinches, grated

cold beetroot and apple soup

Beetroot has been used for centuries by naturopaths for blood and skin disorders. It is extremely rich in betacarotene, which your body converts into vitamin A – one of the most important of all the radiance nutrients.

Put the beetroot and onion into a food processor with half the apple juice and whizz until smooth. Add the rest of the juice, plus the lemon juice and sour cream. Stir well, season to taste with salt and pepper and chill in the fridge until ready to serve.

beetroot	500g, uncooked, peeled and grated
onion	1, finely sliced
apple juice	1 litre
lemon	juice of 1
sour cream	150ml
salt and black pepper	to season

greek salad

tomatoes	250g, quartered
onion	1, finely sliced
green pepper	1, deseeded and cubed
cucumber	1, peeled, deseeded and cubed
black olives	12
feta cheese	125g, cubed
extra-virgin olive oil	75ml
fresh oregano	3 tbsp roughly chopped leaves.

Every mouthful of this salad just bursts with Mediterranean radiance magic . . . lycopene in the tomatoes, vitamin C in the pepper, calcium in the cheese and essential oils in the oregano.

Mix the first 6 ingredients together in a large serving bowl. Drizzle over the olive oil and scatter over the oregano leaves.

broad bean, tomato and herb salad

broad beans	500g shelled weight – fresh are best, but frozen will do
plum tomatoes	4, roughly chopped
extra-virgin olive oil	5 tbsp
fresh oregano	2 tbsp roughly chopped leaves

Cook the broad beans in a saucepan of boiling water until tender. Drain, then pinch off the tough thicker skins unless they're very young and leave to cool. Put the tomatoes into a serving bowl, add the broad beans and mix together. Drizzle over the olive oil and sprinkle the chopped oregano over the top.

aubergine caviar with crudités

aubergines	2 large
lemon	juice of 1
extra-virgin olive oil	3 tbsp
garlic	1 clove, very finely chopped
live natural yoghurt	250g
selection of vegetables– carrots, pepper, celery, cucumber, fennel, cauliflower and broccoli	for the crudités, raw and cut into fine strips or broken into florets

Aubergine provides high levels of radiant and protective anti-oxidants, and the raw vegetables contain skin-nourishing carotenoids, minerals and vitamin C.

Preheat the oven to 200°C/400°F/Gas 6. Put the aubergines into a large roasting dish and bake in the preheated oven until soft, about 20 minutes. Leave to cool slightly then cut open and scrape out the flesh. Put the aubergine flesh into a bowl and add the lemon juice. Gradually beat in the oil and mix in the garlic and yoghurt. Serve as a dip with the raw vegetables.

salad vegeçoise

Radiance on a plate, thanks to the skin-nourishing betacarotene in the peppers, the B vitamins in the eggs and all the natural oils in the olives.

Iceberg lettuce	1, large, roughly shredded
cucumber	½, peeled, deseeded and sliced
red pepper	1, deseeded and cubed
tomatoes	6, quartered and deseeded
eggs	4, hard-boiled and quartered
black olives	12, stoned
my salad dressing (see recipe page 96)	100ml

Put the lettuce into a large, wide bowl. Arrange the other salad vegetables on top. Place the eggs and olives around the side of the bowl. Pour the dressing over the salad and serve.

crudités with garlic mayonnaise

egg yolks	3
garlic	3 large cloves, crushed
salt	a pinch
extra-virgin olive oil	400ml
lemon	juice of 1 small
selection of vegetables— carrots, pepper, celery, cucumber, fennel, cauliflower and broccoli	raw and cut into fine strips or broken into florets

Put the eggs yolks and garlic into a blender with a pinch of salt. Whizz until the yolks are frothy. With the machine still running, add the oil in a fine stream and the lemon juice a little at a time. Transfer to a serving bowl. Serve as a dip with the crudité vegetables.

carrot and melon salad

carrots	3
galia melons	2
sesame seeds	25g
my salad dressing (see recipe page 96)	100ml

Peel and coarsely grate the carrots and peel, deseed and cube the melons. Mix together the carrots and melon. Dry-fry the sesame seeds in a small frying pan until just changing colour. Remove from the heat and leave to cool slightly. Pour over the carrots and melon. Drizzle over the dressing and serve.

puddings

orange soufflé omelette

eggs	4
brown caster sugar	4 tsp
oranges	juice and grated rind of 2
unsalted butter	25g
icing sugar	1 tbsp, for dusting

Separate the egg yolks from the whites. Beat the yolks, then add the sugar, orange juice and rind and mix together. Put the egg whites into a spotlessly clean bowl and whisk into peaks. Fold the egg whites into the mixture. Melt the butter in a non-stick frying pan, pour in a quarter of the mixture and cook the omelette. When it begins to bubble, put the pan under a preheated hot grill to puff up and turn brown. Dust with icing sugar to serve. Repeat to make the remaining omelettes.

fresh fruit brûlée

summer fruits	900g – use thawed frozen fruit if it's the middle of winter
double cream	300ml
live natural yoghurt	250g
brown caster sugar	4 tbsp

All the summer fruits just ooze super nutrients and they are right up there at the top of the inner and outer radiance list. Yes, this is made with double cream – but you aren't going to eat it every day.

Preheat the grill. Put the fruit into a large soufflé dish. Beat the cream, then mix in the yoghurt. Spread the mixture over the fruit and sprinkle the sugar on top. Put the dish under the preheated grill for 4 minutes until the top is golden. Serve immediately.

stewed pears with mascarpone and cloves

firm pears – Conference are ideal	450g, peeled, cored and sliced
sugar	25g
cloves	4
mascarpone cheese	225g

Put the pears gently, sugar and cloves in a large saucepan with 4tbsp of water and cook gently. When they are cooked, remove the cloves and discard. Stir in the mascarpone cheese and leave to cool before serving.

spiced apricots

dried apricots	250g
cloves	4
allspice	½ tsp
apple juice	400ml
runny honey	1tbsp
cinnamon	1 small stick
nutmeg	½ tsp, grated
orange	grated peel of 1

Put all of the ingredients into a large saucepan. Bring to the boil, turn down the heat and simmer until the apricots are tender, about 20 minutes. Remove the cinnamon stick before serving.

pink grapefruit sorbet

caster sugar	200g
rosewater	250ml
pink grapefruit juice	350ml
lemon	juice of 1
pink grapefruit	1, peeled and segmented

Boil the sugar and rosewater for 5 minutes, remove the pan from the heat and leave to cool. Mix with the grapefruit and lemon juice and transfer to a freezing container. Put into the freezer until almost firm. Remove from the freezer, break up with a fork and freeze again. Remove from the freezer 20 minutes before serving and put in the fridge. Serve garnished with the grapefruit segments.

spiced baked apples

ground almonds	2 tbsp
raisins	1 tbsp
orange juice	1 tbsp
cooking apples	4, washed and cored
cloves	4
unsalted butter	50g
brown sugar	1 tbsp
freshly ground nutmeg	4 pinches

It's not just the nutritional value of the apples that's important here, but the anti-bacterial and circulatory-stimulating spices. Together they make this simple pudding a radiance-boosting treat that you can enjoy with a clear conscience.

Preheat the oven to 190°C/375°F/Gas 5. Mix together the almonds, raisins and orange juice. Spoon into the cored cavities of the apples. Top each one with a clove. Use half the butter to grease a large ovenproof dish and the other half to smear over the apple skins. Place the apples in the dish, sprinkle over the sugar and nutmeg and bake in the preheated oven for 25 minutes.

buckwheat crêpes

butter	50g
milk	425ml
buckwheat flour	110g
organic plain flour	110g, sifted
salt	¼ tsp
eggs	4, medium
rapeseed oil	for frying
pumpkin seeds	50g
lemons	the juice of 2 large
runny honey	4 tbsp

Buckwheat isn't, in fact, a cereal; strangely, it's a member of the rhubarb family. So these crêpes are perfect for anyone who genuinely suffers from gluten allergy. It's value in your radiance programme comes from the natural substance called rutin, which strengthens the walls of the tiniest capillary blood vessels under the skin and helps prevent problems like thread veins, spots and other skin blemishes.

Melt the butter and stir it into the milk. Put the flours and salt together in a food processor. Whisking continuously, pour in the milk and butter mixture. Still whisking, add the eggs one at a time until you have a smooth batter. Leave the mixture to rest in the fridge for at least 1 hour.

Brush a crêpe pan or small frying pan with a little oil and heat over a medium heat until the oil is smoking. Pour in a ladleful of batter, tilting the pan to spread it evenly. When the underside is golden, turn the crêpe – or toss it if you feel like showing off – and cook for a further 1–2 minutes. Slide the crêpe onto kitchen paper and keep warm while you repeat with the rest of the batter.

Dry-fry the pumpkin seeds for 2 minutes, until just turning colour. Drizzle each crêpe with the lemon juice and honey, fold in half and serve with the pumpkin seeds scattered on top.

apricot and almond crumble

unsalted butter	50g, cut into small cubes
apricots	50g, stoned and halved
demerara sugar	2 tbsp
porridge oats	175g
ground almonds	50g
runny honey	1 tbsp
flaked almonds	75g

Don't feel guilty about enjoying this delicious pudding. After all, feeling good is a major factor in looking good, and enjoyment of any sort helps you feel good. On top of that, apricots are a major source of vitamin A, almonds provide vitamin E and essential minerals, and oats are rich in the B vitamins. So this is a really sweet treat.

Preheat the oven to 200°C/400°F/Gas 6. Use about half the butter to grease a pie dish. Add the apricots, sugar and 2 tbsp of water. Mix the oats and ground almonds together in a bowl and sprinkle over the top. Drizzle with the honey. Scatter over the flaked almonds and dot with the rest of the butter. Bake in the preheated oven for 20 minutes.

fresh cherry tarts

ready-made puff pastry	1 sheet
fresh cherries	450g, stoned
eggs	2
live natural yoghurt	250g
caster sugar	2 tbsp
cherry brandy	2 tbsp

As well as skin-nourishing protective antioxidants and masses of vitamin C, cherries contain substantial quantities of bio-flavonoids, which slow down the ageing process of the skin.

Preheat the oven to 220°C/425°F/Gas 7. Grease 4 individual loose-bottomed tart tins, roll out the pastry, divide into 4 and use to line the tart tins. Put the cherries on top of the pastry. Beat the eggs together in a bowl. Put the yoghurt, half the sugar and the cherry brandy into a bowl and beat in the eggs. Pour the mixture into the tins, scatter the remaining sugar on top and bake in the preheated oven for 25 minutes, or until the filling has risen and turned a golden colour..

index

picture credits

1 Gettyimages/V.C.L./Paul Viant; 2-3 Gettyimages/Andrea Booher; 4-5 Gettyimages Laurence Monneret; 14-15 Gettyimages/Mark Wright; 17 Gettyimages/Dennie Cody; 20 Digital Vision; 24-25 Gettyimages/John Burwell; 27 Digital Vision; 31 Gettyimages/Szczepaniak; 37 Gettyimages/Jeri Gleiter 43 Digital Vision; 44-45 Gettyimages/Stewart Cohen; 46Gettyimages/ Adrian Neal; 49 Gettyimages/Alan Powdrill; 50 Digital Vision; 55 Gettyimages/Michelangelo Gratton; 56 Gettyimages/Candice Farmer; 68-69 Gettyimages/Scott Morgan; 70-71 Gettyimages/David Rosenberg; 74 Gettyimages/V.C.L./Paul Viant.

acknowledgements

Three years ago our farmer pal. Malc, asked if he could put four of his Highland cattle in our field for a couple of months. Happily for my wife, Sally, and me, these magnificent long-haired, long-horned and placid animals are still there. They've now been joined by Big Bill, a gorgeous Hereford bull, to whom this series of detox books is dedicated.

Bill is the epitome of health, energy and radiance. He's immensely strong, boundlessly active, and his wonderful mahogany-coloured coat has the feel and texture of the finest silk.

Whether you're reading Super Health Detox, Super Energy Detox or Super Radiance Detox, you could all learn from Bill. He lives in an organic field, where he eats what nature intended for him – natural grasses, wild flowers and herbs – which provide all his essential nutrients. If we all lived a little closer to nature, we'd all be healthier, more energetic and more radiant.

I have to thank Sally for her tireless efforts with the recipes, and everyone at Quadrille for the beautiful design of this book. Special thanks must go to Hilary Mandleberg for her understanding, insight and incredible patience.

Editorial Director: Jane O'Shea
Consultant Art Director: Françoise Dietrich
Art Editor: Rachel Gibson
Project Editor: Hilary Mandleberg
Production: Nancy Roberts

First published in 2003 by
Quadrille Publishing Limited
Alhambra House
27–31 Charing Cross Road
London WC2H 0LS

British Library Cataloguing-in-Publication Data
A catalogue record for this book is available from the British Library.

ISBN 1 844000 11 7
Printed in Spain